The Essential Guide to Vitamins Minerals & Supplements

Dr Sarah Brewer

Acknowledgements

I would like to thank everyone who has been so helpful in providing research papers and information on the many invaluable nutritional supplements covered in this book.

Dr Sarah Brewer

Sarah Brewer's first love is medicine and her major passion is writing. She graduated as a doctor from Cambridge University in 1983. She was a full time GP for five years and now works in hospital medicine.

Sarah writes widely on all aspects of health including complementary medicine and is a recognised expert on supplementation.

She has written over 35 popular health books as well as writing for national newspapers and magazines. Sarah was recently voted Health Journalist of the Year.

As well as resident doctor for a number of internet sites, Sarah also regularly appears on television and radio.

Advice to Readers

This book provides useful information on vitamins, minerals and supplements. Every effort has been made to ensure that the contents of this book are accurate and current, but medical and nutritional knowledge are constantly advancing.

This book is not intended to replace medical advice. You should always consult your doctor before taking any nutritional supplements if you are already taking medicines prescribed by your doctor, if you have an illness, or if you think you might be pregnant.

Contents

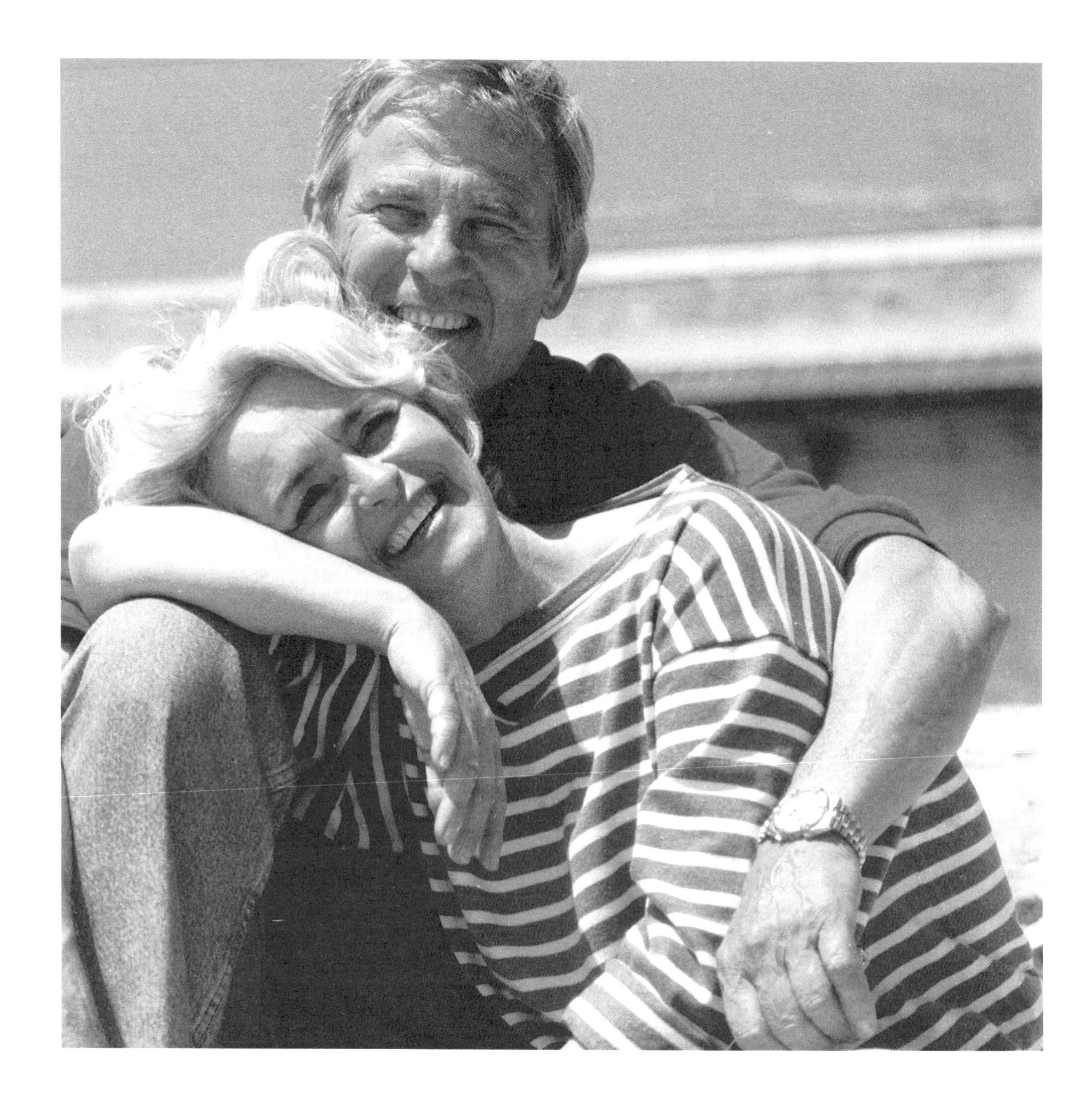

Section One: Essential Nutritional Information

Why food supplements are needed to help maintain optimum health

In an ideal world, we would all get the vitamins, minerals and essential fatty acids we need from our food. In reality, however, few of us achieve this. Three quarters of women and almost nine out of ten men eat less than the recommended five servings of fruit and vegetables per day. In addition, over two thirds of people do not eat oily fish on a regular basis even though one or two portions per week are important for their essential fatty acid content.

Even where average intakes seem satisfactory, it is important to remember that an average is only an average. Where 50% of the population are getting more than the recommended nutrient intake, half may be getting less.

Vitamin and mineral deficiency

Most of our metabolic enzymes (needed to speed chemical reactions occurring in the body) need vitamins, minerals or co-enzymes to function properly. If an essential micronutrient is lacking, vital regeneration and repair processes will slow down *(See table 1)*.

It's estimated that 60% of the population do not obtain 60mg vitamin C on a regular basis. Even more - over 90% of the population - do not obtain the recommended 10mg vitamin E. We don't yet have a recommended daily amount for carotenoids, but a minimum intake of 6mg per day (equivalent to 100ml carrot juice) appears to protect against cancer and age-related macular degeneration. Most of us get less than 2mg carotenoids daily from our food.

On top of this, increasing evidence suggests that higher intakes of these important antioxidants might give significant benefits. Those with the highest intakes of vitamins C, E and carotenoids are less likely to develop coronary heart disease, cataracts, chronic inflammatory diseases and even cancer. As a result, the US Food and Nutrition Board recently recommended an increase in the US Recommended Dietary Allowance (RDA) of vitamin C from 60 to 120mg/day – twice that currently recommended in the UK. Some experts are now advocating daily intakes of 250mg vitamin C, 30-50mg vitamin E and 10 - 15mg carotenoids for optimal health. Although diet should always come first, it is difficult to maintain these high levels of intake without taking a good quality food supplement as a nutritional safety net.

The situation with minerals is even worse. Even when the lowest possible intake of a mineral (LRNI - the amount necessary to prevent deficiency disease) is used as a baseline, government surveys suggest that in women aged 19 to 50 years 10% do not even obtain the LRNI for calcium, 26% do not get the LRNI for iron, 13% do not reach the LRNI for magnesium and 27% do not obtain the LRNI for potassium. Figures for teenagers are significantly worse.

Table 1: Vitamin and mineral deficiency

Most of our metabolic enzymes need vitamins, minerals or co-enzymes to function properly. If an essential micronutrient is lacking, vital regeneration and repair processes will slow down to cause, for example:

- poor wound healing and easy bruising with vitamin C or zinc deficiency
- scaly skin and inflamed gums when vitamin A is in short supply
- nerve problems with vitamin B1 deficiency
- mouth ulcers, sore tongue or cracked lips seen with lack of vitamin B2, vitamin B3, vitamin B6, vitamin B12, folic acid, vitamin C or iron
- premature wrinkles seen in vitamin B3 or selenium deficiency
- disc and cartilage problems in manganese deficiency.

And that's just for the lower reference nutrient intake. When you consider that optimum intakes of calcium are at least 800 - 1000mg per day, and that menstruating women ideally need at least 14mg iron per day, the number of women obtaining less than optimal levels of minerals is staggering.

Vegetarians

Most experienced vegetarians know exactly what constitutes a healthy diet, and many also take supplements. New vegetarians who simply cut out meat without substituting pulses, wholegrains and alternative protein sources are at risk of nutrient deficiency. In particular, intakes of vitamin B12, iron, calcium and zinc need to be watched.

Slimmers

Slimmers are at special risk of vitamin and mineral deficiencies. As food intake decreases, so does the amount of micronutrients obtained. Food surveys suggest that, compared to non-slimmers, dieters on average obtain less vitamins and minerals *(See table 2)*.

For nutrients marked with a double asterisk, the average slimmer does not even obtain the recommended daily amounts.

Although diet should always come first, it is difficult for a slimmer who is cutting back on food and energy intake, increasing their level of exercise and burning excess fat, to get all the vitamins and minerals they need from food alone. Most nutritional experts now agree that a vitamin and mineral supplement is vital when losing weight.

A Healthy Diet

It is possible to get all the nutrients you need from your diet, but unless you are eating the following recommended amounts, your intake of essential fatty acids, vitamins and minerals is likely to be low *(See table 3)*.

Taking a good quality supplement seems an increasingly good idea.

Essential fatty acids

Essential fatty acids (EFA) are oils that are vital for the smooth functioning of the body. They act as building blocks for cell membranes and sex hormones and are vital for healthy nerves and skin. Although your body can make small quantities of essential fatty acids, it cannot produce enough to meet your needs. They must therefore come from eating nuts, seeds and vegetable oils such as linseed and rapeseed oil products. Although the body can make do with the next best fatty acid if an essential one is in short supply, this can lead to common problems such as dry, flaking, itchy skin, cyclical breast pain and pre-menstrual syndrome. Supplements containing evening primrose and starflower oils are therefore growing in popularity.

Although oily fish are so good for health, they can contain pollutants such as dioxin and polychlorinated biphenyls (PCBs). As a result, some guidelines suggest eating no more than

Table 2: Slimmers

For nutrients marked with a double asterisk, the average slimmer does not even obtain the recommended daily amounts.

** vitamin A	* vitamin C
* betacarotene	** vitamin D
** vitamin B1	** vitamin E
** vitamin B2	** iron
* vitamin B3	** calcium
** vitamin B6	** copper
* vitamin B12	** iodine
** folate	** magnesium
* biotin	** zinc

Table 3: A Healthy Diet

- five servings of fresh fruit and vegetables per day (not counting potatoes!)
- 30g of pulses, nuts or seeds per day
- two or three servings of fish per week
- at least half your daily calories from unrefined, complex carbohydrates (cereals, wholegrains bread, wholewheat pasta and brown rice)

one portion per week. This makes taking supplements that have been tested and guaranteed to have low levels of pollutants even more important.

Food quality

Food quality is also an issue. Even when you do eat good amounts of healthy foods, their nutritional content is depleted compared with just a few decades ago. Apart from genetic manipulation to obtain produce specially bred for their colour, uniform size and ability to keep their appearance for longer (at the expense of flavour and nutrients), intensive farming practices often mean that the soils in which crops are grown, and on which livestock are reared, are deficient in vital trace elements. The most startling example is selenium - intakes have dropped significantly over the last 25 years, and in Britain have almost halved from 60mcg in 1974 to just 34 mcg per day in 1994. Our intakes of essential fatty acids (found in nuts, seeds and fish) are also low with an estimated eight out of ten adults deficient in EFAs. Deficiency of EFAs during pregnancy is now implicated in the development of dyslexia, attention deficit hyperactivity disorder and even schizophrenia in the resultant offspring.

Foods can be poor in vitamins and mineral content for a number of reasons *(See table 4)*.

If your diet is healthy, contains at least a pound in weight of fresh fruit and vegetables every day (not counting potatoes) and you eat nuts and seeds regularly, you may not need supplements, but remember that food processing removes many of the vital nutrients, and that food must be eaten fresh. A carton of fresh orange juice left open in the fridge will lose most of its vitamin C content within 3 days.

Doctors are doing it

Out of a straw poll of ten doctor friends, 9 admitted to taking supplements themselves on a regular basis. Most took a multivitamin and mineral supplement plus high dose antioxidants. Five out of 10 took standardised garlic powder tablets, 3 (all women) took evening primrose oil supplements per day, while 3 males took both glucosamine and omega-3 fish oils. If doctors are protecting their future health by paying attention to their vitamin and mineral intake, it must have something going for it!

Taking an A to Z style vitamin and mineral supplement providing around 100% of the recommended daily amount (RDA) of as many vitamins and minerals as possible, plus an essential fatty acid supplement (eg evening primrose, flaxseed, hempseed or fish oils) act as a nutritional safety net, and are an increasingly wise investment for all adults.

Over 50's

As you get older, your need for particular vitamins and minerals will change and the amount of nutrients that can be absorbed from your intestines will decrease. It is therefore a good idea to take a vitamin and mineral supplement designed for your age group and several are now specially formulated for those in later life. Research involving 96 older people showed that those taking multivitamins for one year had better immune function, mounted a better

Table 4: Reasons for poor vitamins and mineral content.

- Food staples are grown in artificially fertilised soils boosted with nitrogen, phosphorus and potassium. Other minerals and trace elements present in soil are not replaced unless soil is organically fertilised. This does not interfere with plant growth, but seriously reduces the plant's nutritional benefit to humans.
- Pesticides and other pollutants interfere with nutrient content of plants
- Foods may be shipped from abroad and picked before ripe - nutrient content will then fall rather than increase
- Foods may be heavily processed or pre-packaged for convenience
- Food additives interfere with the nutrient content of prepared foods
- Stored foods rapidly lose their vitamin content
- Cooking foods rather than eating them raw decreases nutrient content - either by destroying it or leaching it into cooking water

response to influenza vaccination, and had half as many days ill with infections compared with those not taking multivitamin supplements (23 days in the year versus 48).

What you need to know about Vitamins

The word vitamin was first used by the Polish chemist Casimir Funk in 1911. He invented the term as a contraction of two words, vital (from vita, meaning life) and amine (a chemical group originally incorrectly thought to be present in all vitamins).

Vitamins are aptly named. They are naturally-occurring micronutrients that are literally essential for life. Because their chemical structure is based on the element carbon, they are classed as organic substances. There are 13 major vitamins that cannot be synthesised in the body - or only in tiny amounts that are too small to meet most peoples needs (eg vitamin D, niacin). They must therefore come from our diet.

Most vitamins are needed as essential intermediaries or catalysts to help keep metabolic reactions running smoothly and efficiently *(See table 5)*.

The saying "you are what you eat" was never more true than for these micronutrients. If intakes of any vitamin are consistently low, the metabolism cannot function smoothly and problems can occur *(See table 6)*.

How quickly these deficiencies cause problems will depend on how quickly the body's store of a particular vitamin runs out. In the case of folic acid, for example, symptoms of deficiency may show within weeks as it is poorly stored. In contrast, the body usually has good stores of vitamin B12, and deficiencies may take years to show up. In general, the more fat-soluble a vitamin, the better the body can store it. Vitamins are therefore classified into two main groups *(See table 7)*.

What you need to know about Minerals

The word mineral literally means "mined from the earth". Minerals can be divided into two main groups, metallic and non-metallic elements. The word mineral is usually used when referring to inorganic substances of which we need to obtain more than 100mg per day from our diet. Those needed in amounts much less than 100mg are referred to as trace elements.

Around 20 minerals and trace elements are essential for the biochemical reactions occurring in human metabolism. The average adult contains around 3kg of minerals and trace elements, most of which are found in the skeleton.

Although some vitamins can be synthesised in the body in tiny amounts, minerals and trace elements can only come from the diet. As a result, mineral deficiency is more common than vitamin deficiency, especially amongst slimmers, the elderly, pregnant women, vegetarians and those eating vegetables grown in mineral-poor soils. This is because the mineral content of foods depends on the soil in which produce is reared or grown. This is in contrast to the vitamin content of food, which is usually similar where-ever it is produced in the world.

Table 5: Metabolic reactions

These reactions include those responsible for:

- converting fats and carbohydrates into energy
- digestion of foods
- cell division and growth
- repair of damaged tissues
- healthy blood
- fighting infection
- mental alertness
- healthy reproduction
- mopping up harmful by-products of metabolism such as free radicals.

Table 6: "You are what you eat"

Problems can occur such as:

- dry, itchy skin
- tiredness and lack of energy
- poor wound healing
- increased susceptibility to infection

Table 7: Two main vitamin groups

- the fat soluble vitamins (A, D, E and K) which can dissolve in fat and can therefore be stored in the body - mainly in the liver
- the water soluble vitamins (B group and C) which dissolve in water, and are easily lost in the urine. These cannot be stored in the body in appreciable amounts (with the exception of vitamin B12) and must therefore be continually replenished from the diet.

Acid rain and food processing can also reduce the mineral content of foods enough to cause deficiency.

Minerals have a number of roles in the body *(See table 8)*.

What you need to know about EC RDAs for vitamins and minerals

Vitamins and minerals are micro-nutrients which, although essential for health, are only needed in tiny amounts. The quantities you need are measured in milligrams (mg) or micrograms (mcg).

1 milligram = one thousandth of a gram (1/1000 or 10^{-3} grams)
1 microgram = one millionth of a gram (1/1,000,000 or 10^{-6} grams)
1 milligram therefore = 1000 micrograms.

The EC Recommended Daily Amount (RDA) for vitamins and minerals is an estimated intake believed to supply the needs of most (up to 97%) of the population. Everyone has different, individual nutrient needs depending on their age, weight, level of activity and the metabolic pathways and enzyme systems they have inherited so some people will need more, and some people will need less. The EC RDAs suggest the following intakes of each vitamin and mineral:

VITAMINS	EC RDA	MINERALS	EC RDA
Vitamin A (retinol)	800 mcg	Calcium	800mg
Vitamin B1 (thiamin)	1.4mg	Iodine	150 mcg
Vitamin B2 (riboflavin)	1.6mg	Iron	14mg
Vitamin B3 (niacin)	18mg	Magnesium	300mg
Vitamin B5 (pantothenic acid)	6mg	Phosphorus	800mg
Vitamin B6 (pyridoxine)	2mg	Zinc	15mg
Vitamin B12 (cyanocobalamin)	1 mcg		
Biotin	0.15mg		
Folic Acid	200 mcg		
Vitamin C	60mg		
Vitamin D	5 mcg		
Vitamin E	10mg		

As food surveys suggest that only 1 in 10 people obtain all the vitamins and minerals they need from their food, more and more people are choosing to take a multinutrient supplement as a nutritional safety net.

Table 8: The role of minerals in the body

- Structural eg calcium, magnesium and phosphate which strengthen bones and teeth
- Maintaining normal cell function eg sodium, potassium, calcium.
- Co-factor for important enzymes eg copper, iron, magnesium, manganese, molybdenum, selenium, zinc
- Involved in oxygen transport eg iron
- Hormone function eg chromium, iodine
- Act as antioxidants eg selenium, manganese

Some trace elements such as nickel, tin and vanadium are known to be essential for normal growth in only tiny amounts, although their exact roles is not yet fully understood.

What you need to know about upper safe levels for vitamins and minerals

While lack of certain vitamins and minerals can cause problems, many are also harmful in excess. Do not exceed the manufacturer's recommended daily intake of any supplement as it is not the case that more is better.

Safe upper limits for many vitamins and minerals have not yet been set, although the following table provides a good guideline:

VITAMINS	UPPER SAFE LEVEL FOR LONG-TERM CONSUMPTION	MINERALS	UPPER SAFE LEVEL FOR LONG-TERM CONSUMPTION
Vitamin A (retinol)	3000mcg	Calcium	1500mg
Vitamin B1 (thiamin)	50mg	Iodine	1000 mcg
Vitamin B2 (riboflavin)	200mg	Iron	20mg
Vitamin B3 (as nicotinamide)	500mg	Magnesium	700mg
Vitamin B5 (pantothenic acid)	1000mg	Manganese	20mg
Vitamin B6 (pyridoxine)	100mg	Phosphorus	1100mg
Vitamin B12 (cyanocobalamin)	3000 mcg	Zinc	30mg
Biotin	2500 mcg		
Folic Acid	1000 mcg		
Vitamin C	1000mg		
Vitamin D	20 mcg		
Vitamin E	750mg		

What you need to know about Antioxidants

An antioxidant is a protective substance that helps to neutralise damaging oxidation reactions in the body – it literally stops us going rancid and rusty inside.

Several essential vitamins and minerals act as antioxidants. These are protective substances found throughout the body, which mop up harmful by-products of the metabolism known as free radicals. The most important dietary antioxidants *(See table 9)*.

What are free radicals?

A free radical is an unstable molecular fragment that carries a minute, negative electrical charge in the form of a spare electron. It tries to lose this charge by passing on its spare electron during collisions with other molecules and cell structures. This process is known as oxidation. Oxidation usually triggers a harmful chain reaction in which electrons are passed from one molecule to another with damaging results.

Table 9: The most important dietary antioxidants are:

- vitamin A and betacarotene
- vitamin C
- vitamin E
- selenium

Lesser antioxidants that are also important include:

- riboflavin
- copper
- manganese
- zinc.

Other antioxidants include pine bark extracts, co-enzyme Q10, carotenoids such as lutein and lycopene, bilberry, ginkgo, green tea and grapeseed extracts.

Body proteins, fats, cell membranes and genetic material (DNA) are constantly under attack from free radicals, with each cell undergoing an estimated 10,000 free radical oxidations per day. These collisions and chain reactions have been linked with *(See table 10)*.

Free radicals are continuously produced in the body as a result of *(See table 11)*.

Antioxidants are the body's main defence against free radical attack. They quickly neutralise the negative charge on a free radical before it can trigger a chain reaction.

Many antioxidant supplements are now available to help quench free radicals and protect against their harmful effects on health.

Although diet should always come first, many experts now agree that food cannot supply the optimum quantities of antioxidants needed. RDAs for antioxidants such as vitamin C were defined as a means of preventing deficiencies such as scurvy, and modern evidence suggests we might benefit from higher intakes. When calculating the daily intake of antioxidant vitamins needed to obtain the same high blood levels as the 20% of people with the lowest risk of coronary heart disease and cancer, the following intakes are obtained:

- Vitamin C 250mg/day
- Vitamin E 100mg/day
- Mixed carotenoids 15mg/day
- Selenium 100mcg/day

People who smoke, who have diabetes and who are on a slimming diet probably need at least twice as many antioxidants as other people.

What you need to know about Essential Fatty Acids

Essential fatty acids (EFAs) belong to a group of oils known as long-chain polyunsaturated fatty acids (LCPs). While your body can make small amounts of the EFAs from other dietary fats, they are often in short supply and must come from the diet in nuts, seeds, green leafy vegetables, oily fish and wholegrains. There are two main EFAs, linoleic acid and linolenic acid.

EFAs act as building blocks to make cell membranes, sex hormones, and hormone-like chemicals (prostaglandins) found in all your body tissues. EFAs can also be converted into two other types of LCPs: arachidonic acid (AA) which you make from linoleic acid, and docosahexaenoic acid (DHA) which you make from linolenic acid.

As many as 8 out of 10 people do not get enough EFAs from their diet, or are unable to synthesise optimal amounts due to excessive intakes of saturated fat, sugar and alcohol, lack of vitamins and minerals, smoking cigarettes or being under excessive stress.

Lack of EFAs has been linked with a wide range of problems from dry, itchy or inflamed skin to hormonal problems such as acne, prostate problems and low sex drive.

Table 10: collisions and chain reactions

- hardening and furring up of the arteries
- coronary heart disease
- deteriorating vision due to cataracts and macular degeneration
- premature ageing of the skin
- chronic inflammatory diseases such as arthritis
- Alzheimer's disease
- Parkinson's disease
- impaired immunity
- poor sperm count and poor sperm quality
- congenital birth defects.
- cancer

Table 11: collisions and chain reactions

- hardening and furring up of the arteries
- normal metabolic reactions
- muscle contraction during exercise
- smoking cigarettes
- drinking excessive amounts of alcohol
- exposure to environmental pollutants
- exposure to x-rays
- exposure to UVA sunlight, especially if sunburned
- taking some drugs - especially antibiotics or paracetamol

When you do not get enough essential fatty acids from your diet, the metabolism can make do with the next best fatty acids available (eg derived from saturated fats) but as a result prostaglandin imbalances are common. This increases the risk of hormone imbalances, dry, itchy skin, chronic inflammatory diseases (eg rheumatoid arthritis, psoriasis and eczema) and gynaecological problems such as cyclical breast pain.

EFAs are especially important in pregnancy, as they are needed for the structure and development of a developing baby's eyes and brain. Studies suggest that male babies have a higher need for EFAs than females, and lack may increase the risk of developmental problems such as attention deficit hyperactivity disorder and dyslexia.

Lack of EFAs during early childhood has been linked with an increased risk of allergies such as eczema, asthma and hayfever in later life, and may also be linked with cradle cap - a scaly scalp condition - in newborn infants.

If you do not eat plenty of nuts, seeds, wholegrains, fish and dark green leafy vegetables, an essential fatty acid supplement (eg evening primrose or omega-3 fish oils) is a nutritionally sound idea.

What you need to know about Herbal supplements

Herbal medicine uses plant extracts for healing. Different parts of different plants are used - roots, stems, flowers, leaves, bark, sap, fruit or seeds depending on which has the highest concentration of active ingredient. Herbal remedies can have powerful effects – between 30% and 40% of prescription drugs are in fact derived from plant origins. In most cases, herbal supplements contain a blend of constituents that have evolved together over thousands of years to achieve a synergistic balance which tends to have a gentler effect than pharmaceutical extracts that contain only one or two ingredients. The risk of side effects with herbal remedies is therefore relatively low.

Herbal extracts are prepared in ways designed to concentrate their active components. Tinctures are made by soaking herbs in an alcoholic base and may be described as, for example, a 1:10 extract, which means that 10% of the tincture is made up of the herbal base, while 90% is solvent.

Solid extracts are prepared by removing the solvent (eg alcohol) and drying the residual solids, which are then powdered to make tablets or capsules.

Solid extracts are described according to their concentration so that, for example, a 10:1 extract means that ten parts crude herb was used to make one part of the extract. The more concentrated the extract, then theoretically the stronger it is, although more volatile components may have become lost so that the concentration does not accurately reflect its activity. Because of this, it is best to select a standardised preparation where possible.

Standardised Herbal extracts

The amount of active ingredients each plant contains varies depending on a number of factors such as its genetic background, the soil in which it is grown, the time of year and methods of cultivation. As the quality of different batches of raw material can vary significantly, standardisation helps to ensure consistency. It ensures that each batch you buy provides consistent amounts of one or more active ingredients and provides the same benefit. Although only one or two ingredients may be assayed to ensure a standardised concentration, this does not, in any way, discount the undoubtedly important synergy that occurs between the other components present, but whose concentration has not been exactly determined. Standardisation is merely a tool that reassures you that your selected product consistently delivers an effective dose. One part of a standardised extract may be prepared from as much as 50 parts dried leaves or more, which is another reason why standardised extracts are so effective. Cheap, non-standardised products may contain little, if any, active components. Standardised remedies are more likely to be backed by good quality, randomised, double-blind, placebo-controlled trials

What you need to know about potential problems when taking supplements with prescription drugs

An estimated 41% of UK adults take some form of supplement, whether vitamins, minerals, fish oils or herbal remedies. One third take them on a daily basis. Sales of supplements have doubled in the last 4 years, and look set to increase with a steady growth of 13% estimated over the next 4 years.

The number of prescriptions for orthodox medications is also increasing, and many people taking a food supplement or herbal remedy will also be taking at least one prescribed drug. In fact, the popularity of complementary medicine has now increased to the extent that 30% of people use them at the same time as conventional medications. Although the risk of a serious interaction is low, and many potential interactions are theoretical, an increasing number of herb-drug interactions have now been identified. Occasionally, an interaction is severe enough to cause the herb's withdrawal from the market, as was the case with Kava Kava where suspected interactions with alcohol and other drugs may have caused liver damage. It is therefore important that people who wish to take a herbal medicine should ideally check with a pharmacist or doctor if they are taking any orthodox drugs, whether prescribed or obtained over-the-counter.

Unfortunately, surveys suggest that between 47% and 72% of people fail to tell their healthcare professional that they are taking a herbal treatment. And even where someone does check, many pharmacists and doctors do not have information readily to hand, although information on important herb-drug interactions (eg St John's Wort) are sent to doctors and pharmacists by the Medicines Control Agency when appropriate.

Vitamins, minerals and drugs

In general the risk of serious interactions between vitamins, minerals and prescribed drugs is low. Most people can safely take a multivitamin and mineral supplement supplying one or two multiples of the RDAs. In fact, many drugs (eg oral contraceptives) appear to deplete body stores of vitamins and minerals so that supplements seem desirable. Specialist supplements supplying many times the RDA of a particular nutrient need to be checked out on an individual basis, however.

Warfarin seems to be the main drug to be wary of here. Supplements containing vitamin K should be avoided unless directed by a doctor (there are occasions when this interaction is desirable to help reduce the risk of excessive bleeding when taking Vitamin K, but this should only be done under the supervision and advice of the prescribing doctor). High dose vitamin E inhibits platelet aggregation and interferes with vitamin K-dependent clotting factors, so may interact with warfarin, although a clinical trial found no difference in warfarin activity between those taking either vitamin E (up to 1,200mg daily) or placebo. Co-enzyme Q10 is structurally similar to vitamin K and may interact with warfarin activity. Iron magnesium and zinc may bind with warfarin so should be taken at least 2 hours apart from warfarin tablets.

Taking high dose vitamin C (3g) with paracetamol has been shown to prolong the time the drug stays in the body.

Essential fatty acids and drugs

Essential fatty acid supplements such as omega-3 fish oils, cod liver oil, flaxseed oil and evening primrose oils can usually be safely combined with prescription drugs at recommended doses.

Omega-3 fish oils may have anti-clotting activity and may increase the potential for bleeding in people taking warfarin or aspirin.

Herbal remedies and drugs

Interactions occur when a drug and herb act on the same receptor sites in the body, or interact with the same metabolic enzymes. The drugs most likely to interact with herbs are those with a narrow range between the effective and toxic doses, such as anticoagulants, sedatives and some drugs prescribed to treat heart problems, depression, diabetes, high blood pressure and epilepsy.

St John's Wort

The main interactions currently recognised between St John's Wort (Hypericum perforatum) and prescribed drugs are with: warfarin, cyclosporin, oral contraceptives, anticonvulsants, digoxin, theophylline, HIV protease inhibitors used to treat AIDS, and with antidepressants. Most interactions result in reduced blood levels of the prescribed drug. With antidepressants, however, interaction produces an increased effect of serotonin – a brain chemical - which can cause problems. If someone is on any of these medications and taking St John's Wort, they are usually advised to stop the herbal remedy and, if necessary, have blood levels of the drug (eg digoxin) measured in case their drug dose needs adjusting. In one study, for example, St John's Wort decreased absorption of digoxin by 25%, leading to reduced blood digoxin levels.

Warfarin and aspirin and herbs

Warfarin is known to interact with a number of other drugs, and with some herbal remedies. There is also a potential for interaction with herbs that affect the way blood clotting fragments (platelets) stick together, with possible effects on bleeding time, although these are not proven in many cases. These interactions – which may also apply to people taking long-term aspirin *(See table 12)*.

A handful of cases have appeared in the medical literature in which bleeding within the skull (subarachnoid haemorrhage or subdural haematoma) have occurred in people taking Ginkgo biloba extracts in combination with warfarin or aspirin. Although ginkgolides found in Ginkgo biloba do inhibit platelet aggregation, these are present in small concentrations and, at usual therapeutic doses of Ginkgo biloba, effects on platelet aggregation appear to be negligible. However, it may be wiser to err on the side of caution and to avoid using Ginkgo biloba and warfarin until any possible interactions have been fully investigated, although there is no absolute contraindication at present.

If you are taking aspirin and wish to take a herbal remedy, seek advice from a pharmacist who will usually advise you to monitor for bruising or increased bleeding and to seek advice from your doctor if these occur (or will advise that the herbal medication is stopped).

Other notable potential herb-drug interactions some of which are beneficial eg Paracetamol and Milk Thistle (see page 70) *(See table 13)*.

The recognition of interactions – both beneficial and adverse – between herbs, vitamins, minerals and drugs is an evolving area. Information is limited, and often based on single case reports. It is therefore important to always check with your doctor or a pharmacist if wanting to take a supplement together with a prescribed or over-the-counter drug. Most interactions are not serious, but where certain drugs are concerned, it is advisable to err on the side of caution.

What you need to know about the potential benefits of taking a supplement with prescribed medications

Although many people worry about taking food supplements together with a prescribed drug, there are times when this is not only desirable but positively beneficial – either to offset the potential side effects of medication, or to improve its efficacy.

Table 12: Warfarin and aspirin interactions

- Danshen (Salvia species) used to help menstrual irregularity and to relieve bruising
- Dong quai (Angelica sinensis) used to treat menstrual cramps, irregular periods and menopausal symptoms
- Garlic
- Ginseng
- Bilberry
- Chamomile
- Black cohosh
- Ginger
- Pycnogenol (pine bark extracts)
- Red Clover
- Devil's Claw
- Ginkgo

Table 13: Other potential herb-drug interactions

- Diuretics with Dandelion, Ginkgo, Horsetail, Liquorice, Uva-Ursi
- Thyroxine with Lemonbalm
- Paracetamol with Milk Thistle, Schisandra

Antibiotics and probiotics

Probiotics is the use of lactic acid producing bacteria (eg Lactobacilli, Bifidobacteria) naturally found in the large bowel to encourage a healthy digestive balance. Probiotics help to replenish the friendly digestive bacteria that are killed along with the harmful ones when taking antibiotics. This helps to prevent side effects such as diarrhoea and irritable bowel syndrome-like symptoms that can occur when taking antibiotics.

Antibiotics and vitamin K

People taking long-term antibiotics (eg for acne, or because they have had their spleen removed) may benefit from taking a multivitamin and mineral supplying vitamin K. Antibiotics interfere with the action of vitamin K in the body, and also kill probiotic bacteria in the large intestine that produce vitamin K so that levels (needed for healthy blood clotting) are reduced.

Antibiotics and Bromelain

Some evidence suggests that bromelain improves the action of antibiotics (penicillin and erythromycin) in treating a variety of infections. In one trial, 22 out of 23 people who had not previously responded to antibiotics did so once they started taking bromelain as well.

ACE inhibitors and Zinc

The long-term use of the ACE inhibitor, captopril, to treat high blood pressure or heart failure, appears to deplete zinc levels and can lead to a zinc deficiency. It is therefore a good idea for people taking it long-term to also take a multivitamin and mineral supplement that includes zinc.

Paracetamol and Milk Thistle

People taking long-term paracetamol therapy (eg for arthritis pain) may benefit from taking Milk Thistle extracts as well, to help maintain levels of protective glutathione in their liver.

Aspirin, Vitamin C and Zinc

Long term use of aspirin has been associated with increased loss of both vitamin C and zinc in urine, and can lead to vitamin C and zinc depletion. Those on long-term aspirin therapy might benefit from taking supplements providing vitamin C and zinc daily. Non-acidic forms of vitamin C (eg Ester C or other buffered ascorbates) will reduce the risk of acid indigestion).

Antacids, vitamins and minerals

Long term use of antacid can interfere with absorption of nutrients, including folic acid, and possibly copper and phosphate. A multivitamin and mineral supplement is therefore a good idea.

Oral contraceptives, vitamins and minerals

Oral contraceptives appear to deplete body stores of some vitamins and minerals, especially folic acid, magnesium, B1, B2, B3, B6, B12, C and manganese, but may lead to increased levels of iron, and vitamin A. Although the clinical importance of these interactions is unclear, an appropriate folic acid and B group supplement may be sensible.

Statins and Co-enzyme Q10

People taking statins to lower raised lipid (blood fat) levels will experience a significant decline in blood levels of co-enzyme Q10. Supplements supplying CoQ10 are therefore a good idea, and might help to reduce some of the muscle side effects that can occur as a result of statin therapy.

Beta-blockers and Co-enzyme Q10

Betablockers (used to treat high blood pressure and angina) inhibit enzymes that use co-enzyme Q10 as a co-factor. Studies suggest that some beta-blocker-induced side effects (due to propranolol or timolol) can be reduced by taking CoQ10 supplements.

Tricyclic antidepressants and CoQ10

Tricyclic antidepressants interfere with the action of enzymes that use CoQ10 as a co-factor, and it has been suggested that lack of Co-Q10 may contribute to the cardiac side effects of this group of drugs.

SSRIs and Ginkgo

Ginkgo has been shown to help overcome sexual problems which can occur in some people treated with SSRI antidepressants.

Corticosteroids, Calcium and Vitamin D

Long-term corticosteroid therapy is well known to induce osteoporosis. Good intakes of calcium and vitamin D are vital to help maintain bone density and protect against osteoporosis.

Echinacea and topical fungal treatments

One study found that, in women with vaginal Candida, combining oral Echinacea with topical econazole nitrate cream reduced the rate of recurrence compared with those using the anti-fungal cream alone.

What you need to know about buying supplements

A number of supplements are available, as tablets, capsules, powders, pastilles, oils, syrups, teas, infusions, effervescent formulations, tinctures and even gels. As well as the active ingredients, these may contain other substances such as:

Fillers – to increase the volume of material for easier handling

Binders – to cement the substances together so tablets do not crumble

Disintegrants – to help tablets dissolve properly in the digestive tract for optimum absorption

Lubricants – to help the active agents flow during processing

Coatings and glazings – to improve the look and mouth-feel of a tablet so it is easier to swallow.

Capsules – either gelatin or vegetarian–based gels to hold non-tablet ingredients.

In addition, other agents such as colourings, sweeteners, flavourings and preservatives may be used in some cases.

Some tablets are made using a time-release process so the active ingredients are delivered at a steady rate over a longer period of time, usually around 6 hours, rather than all in one go soon after swallowing. This is particularly beneficial for water-soluble vitamins which the body cannot store.

Minerals in tablets are bound (chelated) to other substances, either inorganic salts such as sulphates, carbonates and phosphates or organic substances such as citrates, fumarates, amino acids and ascorbates. This allows them to pass through the stomach without causing irritation, and helps prevent them binding with other substances in the digestive tract which would slow or prevent their absorption. In general, better quality supplements contain minerals bound to organic substances as these are more easily digested and absorbed.

What you need to know about checking labels to assess quality

Deciding what supplements to buy can be confusing as they all seem to offer different benefits at different prices. The labels can help you make your selection, however. The ingredients on the label ingredient box – including the no-active ingredients such as sugar, colourings etc - must be listed in descending order by weight. There will also be a separate nutritional information panel, listing the active ingredients together with their amount and percentage of the RDA where appropriate.

Compare:

The range of nutrients provided in the supplement - is it a complete A to Z type formulation, or does it just provide a few ingredients such as B group vitamins? Does the range of ingredients provided suit your particular needs?

The doses of each nutrient provided – in the case of vitamins and minerals, this will be compared with the recommended daily amount (RDA).

Are minerals chelated with inorganic salts (eg sulphates, carbonates, phosphates) or organic substances (eg citrates, amino acids, ascorbates)? The latter tend to be more expensive, of better quality, and provide greater benefits when taken in supplement form.

Is vitamin E supplied as the natural form, d-alpha tocopheryl, rather than the less active synthetic form, dl-alpha tocopheryl?

The amount of herb provided. Is this included as raw powdered herb or as a concentrated extract? Solid extracts are described according to their concentration so that, for example, a 10:1 extract means that ten parts crude herb was used to make one part of the extract.

Is the preparation standardised to provide a known and consistent quantity of active ingredients? Non-standardised products could contain very little of the key active components.

Does the product suit your particular dietary requirements? For example, is it suitable for vegetarians is it gluten, yeast, lactose or dairy free? Does this matter to you?

Is the product free from artificial sweeteners? Many people prefer to avoid aspartame, for example, especially in children's chewable multivitamin and mineral formulations, although these can be difficult to find!

How does the price relate to the contents of the product?

Check the use by date.

Check who has made it. Is it produced by a well-known, reputable manufacturer whose products are consistently good, and consistently use standardised extracts?

Confusingly, food supplements are not allowed to have health claims on their labels by law. This can make it difficult to know what each particular supplement is designed to do. There may, however, be agreed statements such as: May help to maintain a healthy heart, or May help to replenish the vitamin C lost during colds that provide some useful information to help you select the right product for your needs.

What you need to know about how to take supplements

Vitamin and mineral supplements are usually best taken immediately after food and washed down with water or juice. If taken on an empty stomach, some can make you feel sick or cause indigestion. Don't wash them down with coffee or tea, as these may interfere with absorption. Coffee, for example, reduces iron absorption from the gut by up to 80% if drunk within an hour of a meal. It also reduces uptake of zinc and is associated with increased excretion of magnesium, calcium and other minerals. Against this, however, is the fact that caffeine is a potent stimulator of gastric acid secretion (which will assist absorption of some micronutrients). It is also a rich source of vitamin B3 (niacin) although drinking excess coffee depletes vitamin B levels generally.

If you take a one-a-day vitamin and mineral supplement that is not time released, it is usually better to take it after your evening meal rather than with breakfast. This is because repair processes and mineral flux in your body is greatest at night when growth hormone is secreted. You are also less likely to drink coffee in the evening if it keeps you awake so there is less likely to be a problem with iron absorption.

Where taking two or more capsules of the same preparation a day, its worth spreading these out to maximise absorption and obtain less fluctuating blood levels, assuming this is convenient.

A day's dose is better taken whenever and wherever you remember it however, rather than staying in the packet. Don't feel you have to follow any strict regime if you find difficulty remembering to take supplements, or if they do not fit in with your particular lifestyle.

If you are pregnant or planning to be, or if you are breast feeding, do not take any supplements unless they are specifically designed for use during pregnancy. Always check with a doctor or pharmacist if you are unsure. Some products, such as those containing vitamin A, such as Cod Liver Oil, and most herbs, such as Aloe vera and Agnus castus should not be taken during pregnancy.

Store supplements in a cool, dry place away from direct heat and light.

They should be kept out of the sight and reach of children.

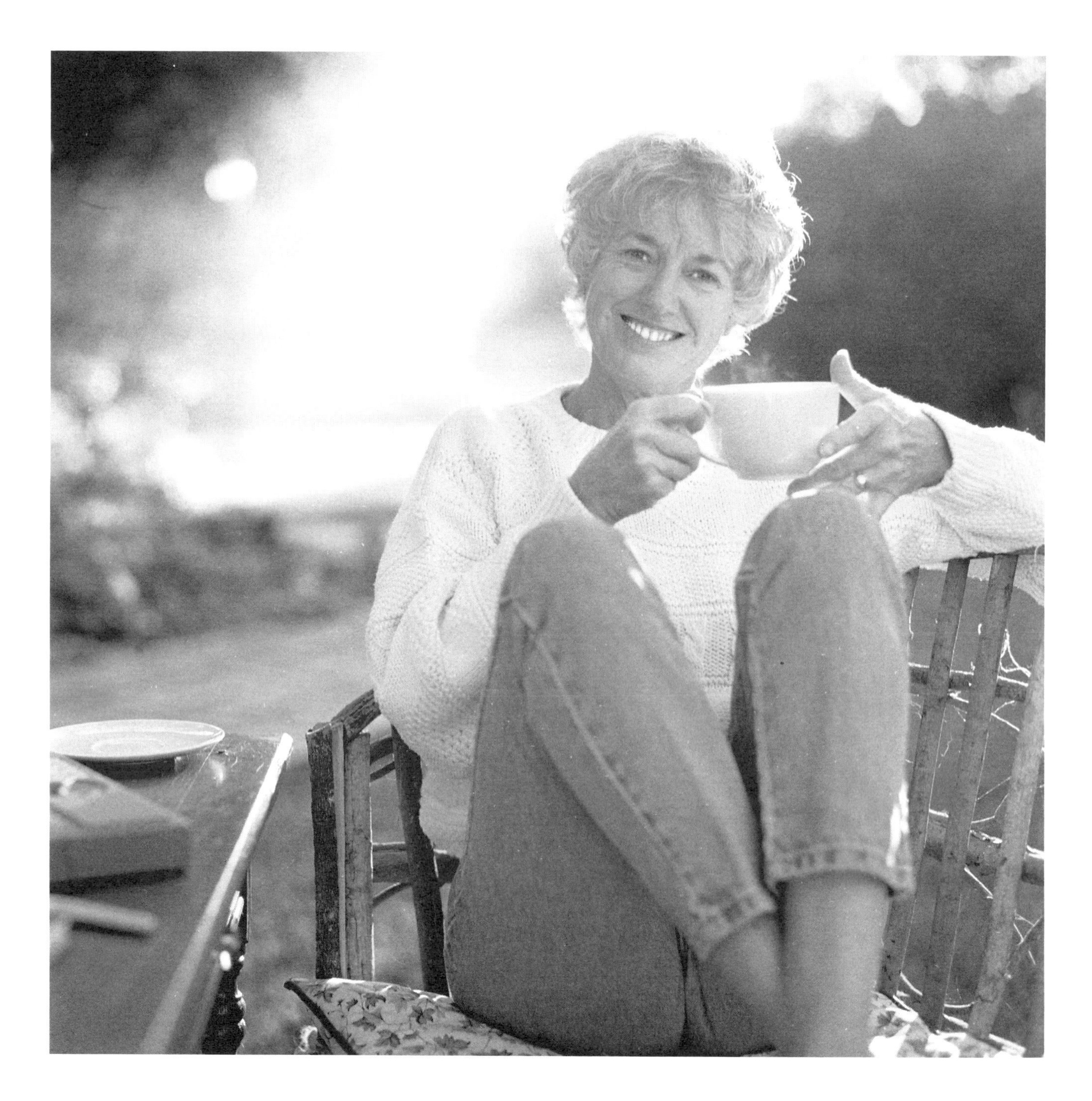

Section Two: The most important Vitamins

Vitamin A (retinol)

WHAT IT IS Vitamin A is a fat soluble vitamin and can be stored in the liver. We obtain vitamin A from two main sources:

- Pre-formed vitamin A (retinol), found only in animal foods
- Carotenoids (mainly betacarotene) which are only found in plant sources *(See betacarotene, page 74).*

WHAT IT DOES Vitamin A is a powerful antioxidant. It also controls genes involved in normal growth, development, healing and immunity, and helps keep the lining of the mouth and lungs moist. In the eye, vitamin A is converted into a pigment, visual purple (rhodopsin) that is vital for vision. When exposed to light, rhodopsin interacts with the back of the eye to trigger messages that are relayed to the brain and interpreted into a series of images.

FOOD SOURCES Foods containing preformed vitamin A (retinol) include:

- animal and fish liver, meat, oily fish and cod liver oil, dairy products, eggs, butter and margarine (fortified by law to contain as much vitamin A as in butter).

Vitamin A is easily destroyed by exposure to light, while betacarotene is destroyed by heat and overcooking. For example:

✖ Boiling or frying reduces vitamin A content by 40% after one hour - by 70% after two hours

HOW MUCH YOU NEED The EC RDA is 800 mcg. Vitamin A is best limited to less than 1,500 mcg per day.

RESEARCH Vitamin A derivatives are available on prescription to treat severe forms of acne, psoriasis and sun damage (photo-ageing) including wrinkles.

SIDE EFFECTS/SAFETY Fat soluble vitamin A readily enters the nervous system and symptoms of retinol poisoning include headache, irritability, blurred vision, nausea, weakness, fatigue. In the long term, excess vitamin A may increase the risk of liver cirrhosis.

High intakes of vitamin A (3000mcg daily or more) during pregnancy may cause certain birth defects. It is advised that pregnant women do not take supplements containing pre-

Symptoms that may be due to minor lack:

- Increased susceptibility to infection
- Scaly skin with raised, pimply hair follicles
- Flaking scalp
- Brittle, dull hair
- loss of sensitivity to green light
- poor eyesight and night vision
- Loss of appetite

Symptoms that may be due to major deficiency:

- Dry, burning, itchy eyes
- Hardening of the cornea
- Eye ulceration

In under-developed countries, half a million people go blind from vitamin A deficiency each year.

formed retinol or eat liver or liver products. As vitamin A is vital for normal healthy development in the womb, however, supplements aimed at pregnant women usually contain carotenoids such as betacarotene (see page 75) that can be converted into retinol when needed. High long-term intakes of 1500 mcg vitamin A may increase the risk of bone fractures.

WHAT TO LOOK FOR WHEN SELECTING A SUPPLEMENT It is best taken in conjunction with other antioxidants such as Vitamins C, E, carotenoids and mineral selenium and zinc.

Do not combine supplements providing vitamin A (eg a multivitamin plus cod liver oil) without checking you are not exceeding recommended levels.

Supplements containing vitamin A are best taken with food as dietary fat aids absorption.

Please note:

- Labels may give amounts of vitamin A as an International Unit (iu)
- 1iu of Vitamin A = 0.3mcg retinol
- 1mcg vitamin A = 3.33iu

B1 (Thiamin)

WHAT IT IS Vitamin B1 is a water-soluble vitamin that is readily lost from the body. Most people only have stores sufficient to last one month. A regular dietary supply is therefore essential.

WHAT IT DOES Vitamin B1 - thiamin - plays a central role in metabolism and the way nerves and muscle cells conduct messages. It is essential for the production of energy from glucose within the body and the more carbohydrate you eat, the more thiamin you will need. It also helps to maintain feelings of calm, alertness and mental energy.

FOOD SOURCES Foods containing preformed vitamin B1 (Thiamin) include:

- Unrefined wholegrains, meat products – especially pork and duck, seafood, fruit, nuts and vegetables, dairy products, eggs, pulses, yeast extract

Thiamin in foods is readily lost during food processing and cooking. For example:

- ✖ Sulphur dioxide, a common preservative in minced meat destroys 90% thiamin content within two days
- ✖ Up to 70% of thiamin content is lost into cooking juices if food is finely chopped or minced
- ✖ Sulphites used to keep processed potatoes white reduce their thiamin content by over 50%
- ✖ Freezing meats reduces thiamin content by up to 50%
- ✖ Cooking meat at 200 degrees C causes a further 20% destruction of thiamin content
- ✖ Baking reduces thiamin content by up to 30%
- ✖ Using baking powder increases losses to 50%
- ✖ Toasting bread reduces thiamin by 10% - 30%

In the UK, white and brown flour are fortified with thiamin to replace losses during production.

HOW MUCH YOU NEED The EC RDA for thiamin is 1.4mg. Older people need to obtain more B1 from their diet to maintain blood levels of this vitamin. Doses of 50mg to 100mg per day may be suggested by nutritional therapists.

DEFICIENCY

Many people over the age of 55 have low dietary intakes of thiamin and those taking diuretics may lose enough thiamin in their urine to cause deficiency.

RESEARCH Vitamin B1 may help reduce symptoms of tingling and numbness that can occur in some forms of nerve disorder such as diabetic neuropathy, multiple sclerosis, Bell's palsy and neuritis.

Taking 10mg vitamin B1 helped people over the age of 65 to enjoy better quality sleep, increased energy levels and lower blood pressure than those taking inactive placebo.

B1 may help to slow the progression of Alzheimer's disease.

SIDE EFFECTS/SAFETY Vitamin B1 is relatively non-toxic as excess is readily lost in the urine. High daily doses (5000mg thiamine hydrochloride or more) may cause headache, nausea, irritability, insomnia, rapid pulse and weakness. These symptoms are reversible once supplements are stopped.

WHAT TO LOOK FOR WHEN SELECTING A SUPPLEMENT

When taking a multinutrient or B complex supplement, check other B group vitamins are also present for optimum value (ie containing B1, B2, B3, B5, B6, B12, biotin and folic acid).

Vitamin B2 (Riboflavin)

WHAT IT IS B2 – riboflavin – is a water soluble vitamin that cannot be stored in the body, so a regular dietary supply is essential.

WHAT IT DOES B2 plays a crucial role in the production of energy and the metabolism of proteins, fats and carbohydrate. People who are physically active need more riboflavin than those who take little exercise. It acts as an antioxidant, is involved in immunity and the production of antibodies and in the formation of hair, skin and nails.

FOOD SOURCES Foods containing preformed vitamin B2 (Riboflavin) include:

Symptoms that may be due to minor lack:

- tiredness
- headache
- loss of appetite
- nausea
- constipation
- irritability
- loss of concentration

Symptoms that may be due to major deficiency:

- depression
- poor memory
- muscle weakness and stiffness
- nerve tingling, burning and numbness
- progressive paralysis

In those with a high alcohol intake, lack of thiamin is associated with Wernicke-Korsakoff syndrome which can lead to irreversible dementia if not corrected.

In underdeveloped countries, thiamin deficiency causes a disease known as beri-beri which means "extreme weakness". Dry beri-beri produces heaviness, weakness, numbness and pins and needles in the legs, while wet beri-beri causes severe fluid retention.

- yeast extract, liver, wholegrain cereals, dairy products, eggs, green leafy vegetables and beans

HOW MUCH YOU NEED The EC RDA is 1.6mg. People who are physically active need more riboflavin than those who take little regular exercise. Older people and those with diabetes need to obtain more B2 from their diet to maintain blood levels of this vitamin.

Intakes of 25mg to 100mg may be suggested by nutritional therapists.

DEFICIENCY Smoking and using the oral contraceptive pill may deplete levels of B2 in the body.

- ✖ B2 is readily lost into cooking water to colour it yellow
- ✖ Light destroys the riboflavin content of milk by 90% after two hours sun exposure – buy milk in cartons rather than bottles
- ✖ Boiling milk reduces riboflavin content by up to 25%.
- ✖ Freezing meat reduces riboflavin by up to 50%.

Symptoms that may be due to minor lack:

- tired, sensitive, gritty, blood shot, red eyes
- mouth ulcers, sores and cracks at the corner of the mouth
- red, inflamed tongue and lips
- scaly eczema-like skin rash, especially on the face and nose
- difficulty sleeping

Symptoms that may be due to major deficiency:

- dull oily hair and hair loss
- split or brittle nails
- trembling
- dizziness
- poor concentration and memory

RESEARCH B2 seems to be important for the brain, as people with good intakes of riboflavin show better scores in tests of mental function than those with low levels.

B2 may be included in supplements designed to improve pre-menstrual syndrome as it is needed to convert vitamin B6 into its active form. It may help reduce migraine attacks, including those associated with menstruation.

B2 has been given together with iron to improve anaemia. It has also been used to help reduce recurrent Candida, carpal tunnel syndrome, cramps during pregnancy and to help cataracts where these conditions are thought to be due to dietary deficiency.

SIDE EFFECTS/SAFETY Excess B2 is excreted in the urine. When taking supplements containing riboflavin, urine colour becomes noticeably more yellow. This is harmless.

WHAT TO LOOK FOR WHEN SELECTING A SUPPLEMENT When taking a multinutrient or B complex supplement, check other B group vitamins are also present for optimum value (ie containing B1, B2, B3, B5, B6, B12, biotin and folic acid).

Vitamin B3 (Niacin)

WHAT IT IS Vitamin B3 - niacin - is a water-soluble vitamin that exists in two forms, as nicotinic acid and nicotinamide. Small amounts of B3 can be made in the body from the essential amino acid, tryptophan.

WHAT IT DOES B3 plays an important role in releasing energy from muscle sugar stores (glycogen) and for processing fatty acids released from body fat stores. It works together with vitamins B1 and B3 to increase energy production in cells, and also works on its own to maintain healthy skin, nerves, intestines and thought processes.

B3, together with mineral chromium, form the Glucose Tolerance Factor (GTF). This is essential for the action of insulin in controlling glucose uptake by cells.

FOOD SOURCES Foods containing preformed Vitamin B3(Niacin) include:

- wheat and maize flour, meat, eggs, milk and yeast extract

In the UK, flour is fortified with B3 to replace that lost during processing.

HOW MUCH YOU NEED The EC RDA is 18mg. People who are physically active need more niacin than sedentary people. Higher doses of 50mg B3 or more per day may be taken for certain medical disorders. Regular blood tests are then usually needed to check liver function.

DEFICIENCY Drinking alcohol may reduce levels of niacin in the body.

RESEARCH B3 is used medicinally to lower abnormally high cholesterol levels. At high doses (under medical supervision) it has been shown to reduce the risk of both non-fatal and fatal heart attacks.

Niacin has also proved helpful in treating hayfever, asthma, depression, arthritis, an overactive thyroid gland, and improving control of blood glucose levels.

SIDE EFFECTS/SAFETY High dose niacin (especially in the form of nicotinic acid) can produce facial flushing. A low dose of aspirin (75mg to 300mg) taken half an hour before B3 can reduce this effect where necessary.

Symptoms of niacin toxicity can occur at very high doses, including thickening and darkening of patches of skin (acanthosis nigricans), palpitations, peptic ulceration, gout, hepatitis and worsening of pre-existing conditions such as diabetes.

WHAT TO LOOK FOR WHEN SELECTING A SUPPLEMENT When taking a multinutrient or B complex supplement, check other B group vitamins are also present for optimum value (ie containing B1, B2, B3, B5, B6, B12, biotin and folic acid).

Supplements may describe their vitamin B3 content in the form of 'niacin' equivalents" which are equal to the amount of nicotinamide and nicotinic acid they contain plus one-sixtieth of their tryptophan content as this can also be converted into B3.

Several supplements were initially called vitamins and given numbers such as B4 but later found not to be essential, so were dropped as vitamins.

Symptoms that may be due to minor lack:

- loss of appetite
- headache
- nausea
- impaired glucose tolerance
- fatigue, weakness
- mouth ulcers

Symptoms that may be due to major deficiency:

- depression
- premature wrinkles
- sore, fissured tongue
- inflamed gut and diarrhoea
- indigestion
- dry, scaly skin in areas exposed to light
- difficulty sleeping
- poor memory
- irritability

In some parts of the world, lack of vitamin B3 produces a rare deficiency disease known as pellagra.

Vitamin B5 (Pantothenic acid)

WHAT IT IS Vitamin B5 - pantothenic acid - is a water soluble vitamin.

WHAT IT DOES B5 is vital for many energy producing reactions in the body involving carbohydrates, fats and protein. It is also necessary for making glucose, fatty acids, adrenal gland hormones, and for maintaining a healthy nervous system.

Vitamin B5 stimulates cell growth in healing tissues, encourages stronger scar tissue formation, helps to rejuvenate ageing skin and to reduce skin mottling. It is also said to improve hair colour and lustre, and to reduce grey hairs.

FOOD SOURCES Foods containing preformed vitamin B5 (Pantothenic acid) include:

- Poultry, meat, offal, wholegrains, eggs, beans and vegetables, especially potatoes and tomatoes, yeast extract

Despite its wide distribution in foods, many people do not get enough pantothenic acid. It is easily destroyed by food processing, for example:

- ✖ Processing wheat reduces vitamin B5 content by 60% if acid or alkaline conditions are present
- ✖ Cooking destroys up to 50% of B5 in meats
- ✖ 30% vitamin B5 in meat is lost into cooking juices
- ✖ Up to 75% of B5 in vegetables is lost during processing
- ✖ Freezing causes a slow destruction of this vitamin

One of the richest supplementary sources of B5 is royal jelly.

HOW MUCH YOU NEED The EC RDA for vitamin B5 is 6mg. Older people may need higher intakes to maintain blood levels of this vitamin.

An intake of around 4mg to 7mg is believed to be adequate, although doses of up to 200mg daily may be suggested by nutritional therapists to treat problems such as chronic fatigue.

DEFICIENCY Vitamin B5 is rapidly depleted during times of stress.

RESEARCH Vitamin B5 derivatives (calcium pantothenate and pantotheine) help to improve liver function in people with viral hepatitis A.

SIDE EFFECTS/SAFETY Very high intakes may cause diarrhoea. Intakes above 100g daily may increase niacin losses in the urine.

Symptoms that may be due to minor lack:

- fatigue
- weakness
- headache
- increased susceptibility to infection
- loss of appetite
- indigestion
- nausea
- difficulty sleeping

Symptoms that may be due to major deficiency:

- poor muscle co-ordination
- muscle cramps
- numbness and tingling
- abdominal cramps
- painful, burning feet
- depression

WHAT TO LOOK FOR WHEN SELECTING A SUPPLEMENT When taking a multinutrient or B complex supplement, check other B group vitamins are also present for optimum value (ie containing B1, B2, B3, B5, B6, B12, biotin and folic acid).

Vitamin B6 (Pyridoxine)

WHAT IT IS Natural vitamin B6 is a group of water-soluble substances that are converted to the active form - pyridoxine - in the body.

WHAT IT DOES Pyridoxine is essential for the proper functioning of over 60 enzymes. It is needed for the synthesis of genetic material, amino acids, proteins and for metabolising body stores of carbohydrate (glycogen) and essential fatty acids.

Regular supplies of vitamin B6 are needed by rapidly dividing cells such as those found in the gut, skin, hair follicles and marrow. It is sometimes called the immune booster as it is needed by cells that produce antibodies and fight infection (lymphocytes). Vitamin B6 is also needed for the synthesis of some brain chemicals and to help regulate the function of sex hormones. It is also necessary for breaking down homocysteine - an amino acid which can increase the risk of coronary heart disease if levels are high.

FOOD SOURCES Foods containing preformed vitamin B6 (Pyridoxine)include:

- whole-grain cereals, meat, especially liver, oily fish, soya products, bananas, walnuts, green, leafy vegetables, avocado, egg yolk and yeast extract.

Vitamin B6 is readily destroyed by cooking and exposure to light.

- ✖ 20% of pyridoxine in milk is destroyed by sterilisation
- ✖ 20% in vegetables is lost by canning
- ✖ 40% is lost into water when frozen vegetables are thawed and cooked
- ✖ up to 70% of vitamin B6 in meat is lost during processing

HOW MUCH YOU NEED The EC RDA for vitamin B6 is 2mg. Higher doses of 100mg to 200mg have been taken to help PMS. Do not take high doses for more than a few months without seeking medical advice.

DEFICIENCY Smoking and taking the oral contraceptive pill may reduce its levels in the body.

Some studies suggest as many as one in five women are deficient in B6.

Symptoms that may be due to minor lack:

- headache
- mild depression
- anxiety
- irritability
- bloating
- tender breasts

These are all common symptoms of premenstrual syndrome.

Symptoms that may be due to major deficiency:

- anaemia
- split lips and recurrent mouth ulcers
- red, inflamed tongue
- burning skin

Lack of vitamin B6 has been linked with carpal tunnel syndrome.

RESEARCH An analysis of 9 trials involving over 900 women suggests that doses of up to 100mg vitamin B6 daily can help reduce symptoms of PMS.

People with chronic fatigue syndrome may be helped by taking B group vitamins, including vitamin B6.

Taking B group vitamins supplements (folic acid plus vitamins B6 and B12) has been shown to lower raised levels of homocysteine to help reduce the risk of a heart attack.

Vitamin B6 supplements can improve memory in older people. They have also been used to improve depression

SIDE EFFECTS/SAFETY There have been some suggestions that prolonged high doses of above 10mg daily may cause reversible nerve symptoms such as pins and needles, but this is controversial. The risks associated with taking vitamin B6 at doses between 10mg and 200mg long term are unclear, but are probably low.

WHAT TO LOOK FOR WHEN SELECTING A SUPPLEMENT When taking a multinutrient or B complex supplement, check other B group vitamins are also present for optimum value (ie containing B1, B2, B3, B5, B6, B12, biotin and folic acid).

Vitamin B12 (Cyanocobalamin)

WHAT IT IS Vitamin B12 is a water-soluble vitamin. It can be stored in the liver, however, and we usually have enough to last several years.

WHAT IT DOES B12 is essential when genetic material (DNA) is synthesised during cell division. When B12 is in short supply, dividing cells become unusually large. When this affects red blood cells, a form of anaemia results. B12 is also needed for healthy nerve function, immunity and healing. Together with folic acid, vitamin B12 protects against some congenital developmental disorders such as spina bifida.

FOOD SOURCES Foods containing preformed vitamin B12 (Cyanocobalamin) include:

- Liver, kidney, meat, oily fish, especially sardines, eggs and dairy products

B12 is only found in animal-based foods in consistent amounts. Supplements supplying synthetic B12, or natural forms derived from blue-green algae or bacterial cultures are available for vegetarians.

✖ around 20% B12 leaches out in juices during cooking

HOW MUCH YOU NEED The EC RDA for B12 is 1 mcg. Intakes as high as 1000 mcg (1mg) per day appear to be safe. Although vitamin B12 supplements to treat pernicious anaemia are traditionally given as regular injections, it can be given orally in very high dose (eg 2mg = 2000 mcg daily).

Alcohol and taking the oral contraceptive pill may reduce body stores of B12.

Symptoms that may be due to minor lack:

- smooth, sore tongue
- tiredness
- exhaustion
- menstrual disorders
- poor memory
- lack of concentration

Symptoms that may be due to major deficiency:

- anaemia
- numbness
- tingling
- trembling
- clumsiness
- difficulty walking, especially in the dark
- confusion
- depression

DEFICIENCY B12 is absorbed in the lower part of the small intestine, but only if a carrier protein, intrinsic factor (made in the stomach) is present. B12 deficiency sometimes develops in later life because of lack of intrinsic factor or disease of the small intestine. Prolonged deficiency leads to symptoms such as pernicious anaemia creeping up slowly. Deficiency that is not corrected can lead to spinal cord damage although this is rare.

RESEARCH Taking B group vitamin supplements (folic acid plus vitamins B6 and B12) has been shown to lower raised levels of homocysteine to help reduce the risk of a heart attack.

B12 has been used to help bio rhythm disturbances (eg jet lag) and vitiligo (loss of skin pigmentation)

SIDE EFFECTS/SAFETY No serious side effects have been reported as excess is excreted in the urine.

WHAT TO LOOK FOR WHEN SELECTING A SUPPLEMENT

When taking a multinutrient or B complex supplement, check other B group vitamins are also present for optimum value (ie containing B1, B2, B3, B5, B6, B12, biotin and folic acid).

Vitamin B12 deficiency can be masked by taking folate supplements so supplements are usually given together.

Biotin

WHAT IT IS Biotin is a water soluble B group vitamin.

WHAT IT DOES Biotin is involved in the synthesis and metabolism of fatty acids, amino acids, genetic material, stress hormones and energy storage molecules such as glucose. It is also essential for healthy hair, skin and sweat glands.

FOOD SOURCES Foods containing preformed Biotin include:

- Meat, liver, oily fish, egg yolk, wholegrains, nuts, cauliflower, yeast extract

HOW MUCH YOU NEED The EC RDA for biotin is 0.15mg (150mcg). For maintaining healthy skin, hair and nails, intakes of around 1mg daily are taken. Two out of three people respond, with nails growing significantly thicker.

DEFICIENCY As biotin is widely distributed in food, and is also made by bacteria in the gut, from which it can be absorbed, dietary deficiency is rare. It can occur in those taking long-term antibiotics, although taking a probiotic supplement containing friendly bacteria (eg Lactobacillus acidophilus) will help to overcome this effect. Biotin deficiency can also occur in body builders who eat large amounts of raw egg white over a long period. Raw (but not

Symptoms that may be due to minor lack:

- dry, flaky skin
- rash around the nose and mouth
- brittle hair and nails
- tiredness
- loss of appetite
- nausea

Symptoms that may be due to major deficiency:

- patches of hair loss (alopecia)
- reversible baldness
- depression
- muscle pains and wasting

cooked) egg white contains a protein called avidin that binds to biotin in the gut and prevents its absorption.

RESEARCH An inherited inborn error of biotin metabolism, which affects around one in 120 people may reduce immunity against yeast infections. Biotin may improve glucose control in people with diabetes.

SIDE EFFECTS/SAFETY No serious side effects reported. Daily intakes of up to 1mg daily appear to be safe.

WHAT TO LOOK FOR WHEN SELECTING A SUPPLEMENT When taking a multinutrient or B complex supplement, check other B group vitamins are also present for optimum value (ie containing B1, B2, B3, B5, B6, B12, biotin and folic acid).

Folic Acid

WHAT IT IS Folic acid is a water soluble vitamin. It is the synthetic, monoglutamate form of the naturally occurring folate (polyglutamate form), and is preferable in supplements as it is more readily absorbed and used more efficiently in the body.

WHAT IT DOES Folic acid is involved in the synthesis and metabolism of proteins, sugar and nucleic acids during cell division. Like vitamin B12, it is especially needed by cells that are dividing rapidly. When folic acid is in short supply, dividing cells become unusually large and, when this affects red blood cells, a form of anaemia results.

Folic acid is essential during the first few weeks of a baby's development in the womb. Deficiency can trigger a type of developmental abnormality known as a neural tube defect (eg spina bifida) which arise between the 24 – 28th day after conception.

FOOD SOURCES Foods containing preformed Folic Acid include:

- green leafy vegetables eg spinach, broccoli, Brussel sprouts, parsley, wholegrains, beans, soya products, liver, kidney, citrus fruit, nuts, dairy products, eggs and yeast extract

Folate is destroyed by prolonged contact with light and air but can be protected by antioxidant vitamin C.

- ✖ up to 90% of folate content of grain is lost during milling
- ✖ 10% of folate in vegetables is lost by steaming, 20% by pressure cooking and up to 50% by boiling.
- ✖ Foods originally rich in folate may have less than one third their folate content left by they time they are eaten.

HOW MUCH YOU NEED The EC RDA for folic acid is 200 mcg. Women planning a baby should take daily supplements containing 400 mcg folic acid (4mg if they have a personal or family history of conceiving a child with a neural tube defect).

High levels of homocysteine can be reduced by taking folic acid supplements (400mcg - 650mcg per day). People with a family or personal history of coronary heart disease may be advised to take at least 400mcg folic acid daily.

The recommended upper safe limit for folic acid is to take no more than 1000mcg daily long-term (unless advised to during pregnancy, for example).

DEFICIENCY The body stores very little folic acid and dietary lack rapidly causes deficiency - it is probably the most widespread vitamin deficiency in developed countries. Drinking excess alcohol may lower folic acid levels.

Symptoms that may be due to minor lack:

- tiredness
- weakness
- irritability
- insomnia
- forgetfulness

Symptoms that may be due to major deficiency:

- anaemia
- muscular cramps
- confusion
- red, sore tongue
- cracking at the corners of the mouth

RESEARCH Taking supplements supplying 400mcg to 4mg folic acid can reduce the risk of spina bifida by over 70%.

Taking B group vitamin supplements (folic acid plus vitamins B6 and B12) has been shown to lower raised levels of homocysteine to help reduce the risk of a heart attack. An intake of 400mg folic acid helps to maintain a healthy heart and circulation.

Low blood levels of folic acid have been linked with an increased risk of Alzheimer's disease.

Research also suggests that folic acid may protect against abnormal cervical smears by encouraging more normal cell division.

People with the skin depigmentation condition, vitiligo, may be treated with folic acid (plus vitamin B12).

People with chronic fatigue syndrome may have low levels of folic acid and there is preliminary evidence that taking B group vitamins (including folic acid) may improve symptoms in some people.

SIDE EFFECTS/SAFETY People taking drugs to treat epilepsy should tell their doctor if they take folic acid supplements - these can interfere with the way their medication works. Women on anti-epileptic drugs should seek medical advice about taking extra folic acid supplements before trying to conceive a baby.

WHAT TO LOOK FOR WHEN SELECTING A SUPPLEMENT When taking a multinutrient or B complex supplement, check other B group vitamins are also present for optimum value (ie containing B1, B2, B3, B5, B6, B12, biotin and folic acid).

Vitamin B12 deficiency can be masked by taking folate supplements so supplements are usually given together.

Vitamin C (Ascorbic acid)

WHAT IT IS Vitamin C - ascorbic acid - is a water soluble vitamin that cannot be stored in the body in appreciable amounts..

WHAT IT DOES Vitamin C is an important dietary antioxidant. It acts as an essential co-factor for at least 300 metabolic reactions which are promoted when large quantities of vitamin C are available. It is essential for the synthesis of collagen, a major structural protein in the body and is necessary for proper growth and repair and for healthy tissues, including bones. Vitamin C is involved in the metabolism of stress hormones and also has antiviral and anti-bacterial actions. Another useful role for vitamin C is its ability to increase absorption of iron – those taking iron supplements for anaemia should ideally wash down their tablets with a glass of orange juice.

FOOD SOURCES Foods containing preformed vitamin C (Ascorbic acid) include:

- blackcurrants, guavas, kiwi fruit, citrus fruit, mangoes, green peppers, strawberries, green sprouting vegetables eg broccoli, sprouts, watercress, parsley and potatoes
- Animal sources include kidney and liver.

Vitamin C is one of the most unstable vitamins and up to two thirds is lost by processing, prolonged cooking and storage. For example:

- ✖ Processing soft fruits loses over two thirds of their vitamin C content
- ✖ Once fruit juices are opened, their vitamin C content rapidly deteriorates, even if chilled - virtually all is lost within 14 days
- ✖ Boiling vegetables loses up to 50% of vitamin C into water
- ✖ Storage of root vegetables loses around 10% of vitamin C content per month
- ✖ Storage of some vegetables (eg asparagus) reduces their vitamin C content by up to 90% after just one week

HOW MUCH YOU NEED The EC RDA for vitamin C is 60mg, although this is widely thought to be too low. The US RDA for vitamin C was recently raised from 60 to 120mg.

Many experts now feel intakes of 500mg to 1g vitamin C daily are optimal. Short term higher intakes (eg 3g daily for the duration of a cold) do not appear to be harmful.

Smokers and those with diabetes mellitus need twice as much vitamin C as non-smokers.

DEFICIENCY Lack of vitamin C causes scurvy. A minimum daily intake (LRNI) of 10mg vitamin C is needed to prevent this - although 20mg per day is needed for proper wound healing.

Symptoms that may be due to minor lack:

- Frequent colds and other infections
- Lack of energy
- Weakness
- poor wound healing
- dry, rough, scaly skin
- broken thread veins in skin around hair follicles
- scalp dryness
- irritability
- muscle and joint pain

Symptoms that may be due to major deficiency:

- misshapen, tangled, brittle hair
- hair loss
- dry, fissured lips
- easy bruising
- loose teeth
- inflamed, bleeding gums,
- bleeding skin, eyes and nose
- depression

RESEARCH Studies show that high intakes of vitamin C (1g daily or more) can halve the severity of symptoms due to the common cold, and reduce the duration of a cold by 20%. For some groups of people – eg athletes, students – it has also been shown to lower the risk of infection after exposure to the cold virus. It seems that viruses cannot reproduce properly in cells with high levels of vitamin C.

The level of vitamin C found in the eye lens is 60 times that found in the circulation. In one study, it was found that those taking 300mg vitamin C daily were 70% less likely to develop cataracts than similar patients not taking supplements.

A ten-year study involving 11,000 people has shown that men with the highest intakes of vitamin C have a 40% lower risk of developing coronary heart disease and a 35% lower risk of dying from it. For women with the highest intakes of vitamin C, there was a 25% lower risk of coronary heart disease. They were also up to 42% less likely to die from cancer. Vitamin C protects cholesterol in the blood stream from oxidation. As only oxidised cholesterol is linked with hardening and furring up of the arteries (atherosclerosis) this is the most likely explanation for why vitamin C protects against heart attack and possibly stroke. It also protects genetic material from oxidation and mutation, which is probably why it seems to protect against cancer.

People with asthma may have reduced symptoms and improved breathing when taking 1g to 2g vitamin C daily.

Vitamin C may reduce the risk of cartilage loss and disease progression in people with osteoarthritis.

A recent study of 19,196 adults aged 45 to 79 years in the UK found that circulating levels of vitamin C were inversely related to death from all causes over the 4 year study period.

SIDE EFFECTS/SAFETY The safety of vitamin C supplementation has been researched and established over a long period of time. Claims that large doses could trigger kidney stones have proved unfounded. However, those known to be recurrent stone formers and people with renal failure who have a defect in ascorbic acid or oxalate metabolism, should restrict daily vitamin C intakes to approximately 100mg.

Taking larger doses may trigger indigestion or diarrhoea, which settles when the dose is reduced. Taking vitamin C in the form of buffered, non-acidic, mineral ascorbates may reduce these problems. Interestingly, when you are ill your vitamin C needs seem to increase to such an extent that you become much more tolerant of high doses so you can take much higher amounts before developing loose bowel motions.

If taking high doses of vitamin C and you need to have a urine or stool test, inform your doctor that you are taking a high dose supplement as it can affect laboratory results.

Individuals with iron-storage disease (eg haemochromatosis) should not take vitamin C supplements except under medical advice.

Those choosing to take very high dose supplements should reduce their vitamin C intake slowly over a few weeks rather than stopping suddenly.

WHAT TO LOOK FOR WHEN SELECTING A SUPPLEMENT To achieve a high intake, vitamin C is best taken spread over several doses per day. Products combining vitamin C with bioflavonoids are better absorbed and provide additional antioxidant benefits.

If choosing a chewable formulation, you may prefer to select one that is free from aspartame.

Vitamin D (Cholecalciferol)

WHAT IT IS Vitamin D is a fat soluble vitamin that can also be broken down in the body to form a hormone (calcitriol).

WHAT IT DOES Vitamin D is essential for the absorption of dietary calcium and phosphate in the small intestine. It therefore plays an important role in maintaining healthy bones and teeth.

FOOD SOURCES Vitamin D can be synthesised in the body by the action of sunlight on a cholesterol-like molecule in the skin. Blood levels of vitamin D are therefore naturally higher in the summer and lower in winter. People living in high altitudes, who cover up their skin in sunlight, or who stay indoors all day are not exposed to enough sunlight to meet their vitamin D needs. They must then rely on getting vitamin D from their diet.

Foods containing vitamin D include:

- oily fish (sardine, herring, mackerel, salmon, tuna), *(the best levels of vitamin D are found in fresh rather than tinned fish)*, fish liver oils, fortified margarine, liver, eggs, fortified milk and butter

HOW MUCH YOU NEED The EC RDA for vitamin D is 5mcg. People over the age of 50 usually need at least double this amount (10mcg) as blood levels fall with increasing age. Intakes of up to 25mcg daily are not thought to be harmful.

DEFICIENCY If vitamin D is lacking during childhood, deformed bones (rickets) result. In adults, weakened, softened bones (osteomalacia) develop. Bone thinning (osteoporosis) in later life can also depend on vitamin D intakes as, when it is in short supply, less calcium is absorbed from the gut. Four out of five people with osteoporotic hip fractures have evidence of vitamin D deficiency.

RESEARCH In a study of postmenopausal women with low vitamin D levels, increasing intakes to 500iu daily (12.5mcg) for one year significantly reduced bone loss in late winter

Symptoms that may be due to minor lack:

- constipation
- muscle weakness
- irritability
- increased susceptibility to infections

Symptoms that may be due to major deficiency:

- poor growth
- bone pain
- bone deformities (in rickets)
- deafness (in osteomalacia)

and increased bone density in the spine. Giving both calcium and vitamin D supplements reduces the risk of hip fracture by up to 40%.

Vitamin D derivatives are used medically to treat some forms of psoriasis.

SIDE EFFECTS/SAFETY Excess vitamin D is toxic and can lead to headache, loss of appetite, nausea, vomiting, diarrhoea or constipation, palpitations and fatigue. Doses above 50mcg may cause problems if taken long-term, although some people are sensitive to lower doses of 25-50mcg daily, which can increase the risk of calcium kidney stones in those who are susceptible.

What to look for when selecting a supplement

Sometimes the amount of vitamin D is expressed in International Units (iu) rather than micrograms. 1mcg vitamin D = 40iu.

Vitamin E (d-alpha-tocopherol)

WHAT IT IS Vitamin E - tocopherol - is a group of 8 fat soluble vitamins. The most active form is natural source d-alpha-tocopherol.

WHAT IT DOES Vitamin E mainly acts as an antioxidant protecting body fats from oxidative damage and rancidity. It has a strengthening effect on muscle fibres (relieving muscle cramps), boosts the immune system and improves skin suppleness and healing.

Selenium and vitamin E have a synergistic effect in antibody synthesis and supplements of both have been found to increase antibody synthesis 30 fold as well as improving the response to influenza vaccinations. Vitamin C is needed to regenerate vitamin E when it has carried out its antioxidant function.

FOOD SOURCES Foods containing Vitamin E (d-alpha-tocopherol) include:

- wheatgerm oil, avocado pear, butter and margarine, wholemeal cereals, nuts and seeds, oily fish, eggs and broccoli.

Fresh raw foods and supplements are the best sources.

- ✖ Rapidly lost by exposure to air
- ✖ Even when frozen, foods can lose up to 70% of their vitamin E content within 14 days
- ✖ Processing cereals and grains removes over 90% of their vitamin E content
- ✖ Frying or roasting will destroy virtually all vitamin E content of food
- ✖ Boiling loses a third of the vitamin E content of vegetables
- ✖ Canning increasing losses by up to 80%

HOW MUCH YOU NEED The EC RDA for vitamin E is 10mg (15iu). Vitamin E supplements usually provide 100iu (67mg), 200iu (134mg) or 400iu (268mg).

Doses of up to 727mg (800 iu/day) supplemental vitamin E may be taken long-term with no apparent ill effects. In general, the more polyunsaturated fats you eat, the more vitamin E you need.

DEFICIENCY

Lack of vitamin E has a harmful effect on the nervous system.

Symptoms that may be due to minor lack:

- lack of energy
- lethargy
- poor concentration
- irritability

Symptoms that may be due to major deficiency:

- lowered sex drive
- muscle weakness

RESEARCH Vitamin E seems to improve glucose balance in the body, and helps people with diabetes to develop a better response to insulin hormone.

A study of over 11,000 people aged 67 years and over found those taking vitamin E had a reduced risk of death at any age by around a third compared with those not taking vitamin E supplements. Risk of death from coronary heart disease was reduced by 63%, risk of death from cancer reduce by 59%. These results took account of other factors such as alcohol use, smoking history, aspirin use and known medical conditions.

In the Cambridge Heart Antioxidant Study (CHAOS) involving over 2000 people with coronary heart disease, taking vitamin E (400 or 800iu daily = 268mg or 536mg) was found to reduce the risk of a heart attack by 77%. Not only was the difference highly statistically significant, it seemed the group treated with vitamin E were at no greater risk of a heart attack than people without coronary heart disease.

Other studies have shown that vitamin E is beneficial in the prevention or treatment of peripheral vascular disease, lung disease, cataracts and neurological problems such as Parkinson's Disease and epilepsy. It also seems to protect against some cancers.

A recent review of over a dozen studies involving centenarians found that vitamin E could be the key to their longer life – healthy people who survive into their 100s appear to have exceptionally high blood levels of vitamin E compared with those found in younger adults!

SIDE EFFECTS/SAFETY High intakes of vitamin E can be toxic (causing headache, fatigue, gastrointestinal distress, double vision, muscle weakness) but this only usually occurs at doses 3000mg daily.

WHAT TO LOOK FOR WHEN SELECTING A SUPPLEMENT High dose vitamin E is best taken together with other antioxidants, such as vitamin C, mixed carotenoids and selenium.

The vitamin E content of foods and supplements is usually expressed in terms of alpha-tocopherol equivalents. Synthetic alpha-tocopherol (dl-alpha tocopherol) has less biological strength (between 36% and 50%) than natural source vitamin E (d-alpha tocopherol) due to the different symmetries of the molecules present.

Select supplements containing natural or natural source vitamin E (d-alpha tocopherol) for their greater bioactivity.

Sometimes the amount of vitamin E is expressed in International Units (iu) rather than milligrams. 1iu= 0.67mg alpha-tocopherol equivalents or conversely: 1mg = 1.5iu

Vitamin K

WHAT IT IS Vitamin K activity is found in a group of four, fat soluble substances: phyllo-quinone (K1), menaquinones (K2), menadione (K3) and menadiol (K4).

WHAT IT DOES Vitamin K is essential for making important blood proteins involved in blood clotting. Vitamin K is also needed for the synthesis of osteocalcin - a calcium-binding protein found in bone.

FOOD SOURCES Most of our vitamin K requirements are met by beneficial bacteria in our gut which produce vitamin K2 which is then absorbed into our circulation

Dietary sources supply around a fifth of our needs, from:

- cauliflower (the richest source), dark green leafy vegetables (eg broccoli, kelp), yoghurt and safflower, rapeseed, soya and olive oils

HOW MUCH YOU NEED No EC RDA for vitamin K is currently set, but requirements are thought to be around 1mcg per kilogram of body weight per day. Supplements oftensupply 10mcg to 300mcg. Higher doses may be suggested for treating osteoporosis. It is thought that a daily supplementary intake of 1mg is unlikely to cause harm.

DEFICIENCY Lack of vitamin K leads to blood clotting disorders.

A single dose of vitamin K is offered to all newborn infants to prevent a condition known as haemorrhagic disease of the newborn. This arises during the first few days of life and causes haemorrhage into the brain due to vitamin K deficiency.

Symptoms due to major deficiency:

- prolonged bleeding
- easy bruising
- recurrent nose bleeds
- heavy periods
- diarrhoea.

RESEARCH Lack of vitamin K has been linked to osteoporosis and, research suggests vitamin K supplements can reduce loss of bone calcium in post-menopausal women by up to 50% and can also strengthen bones that are already weakened.

SIDE EFFECTS/SAFETY Seek medical advice before taking supplements containing vitamin K if you are on warfarin or other blood thinning treatment.

WHAT TO LOOK FOR WHEN SELECTING A SUPPLEMENT Best taken with meals for optimum absorption.

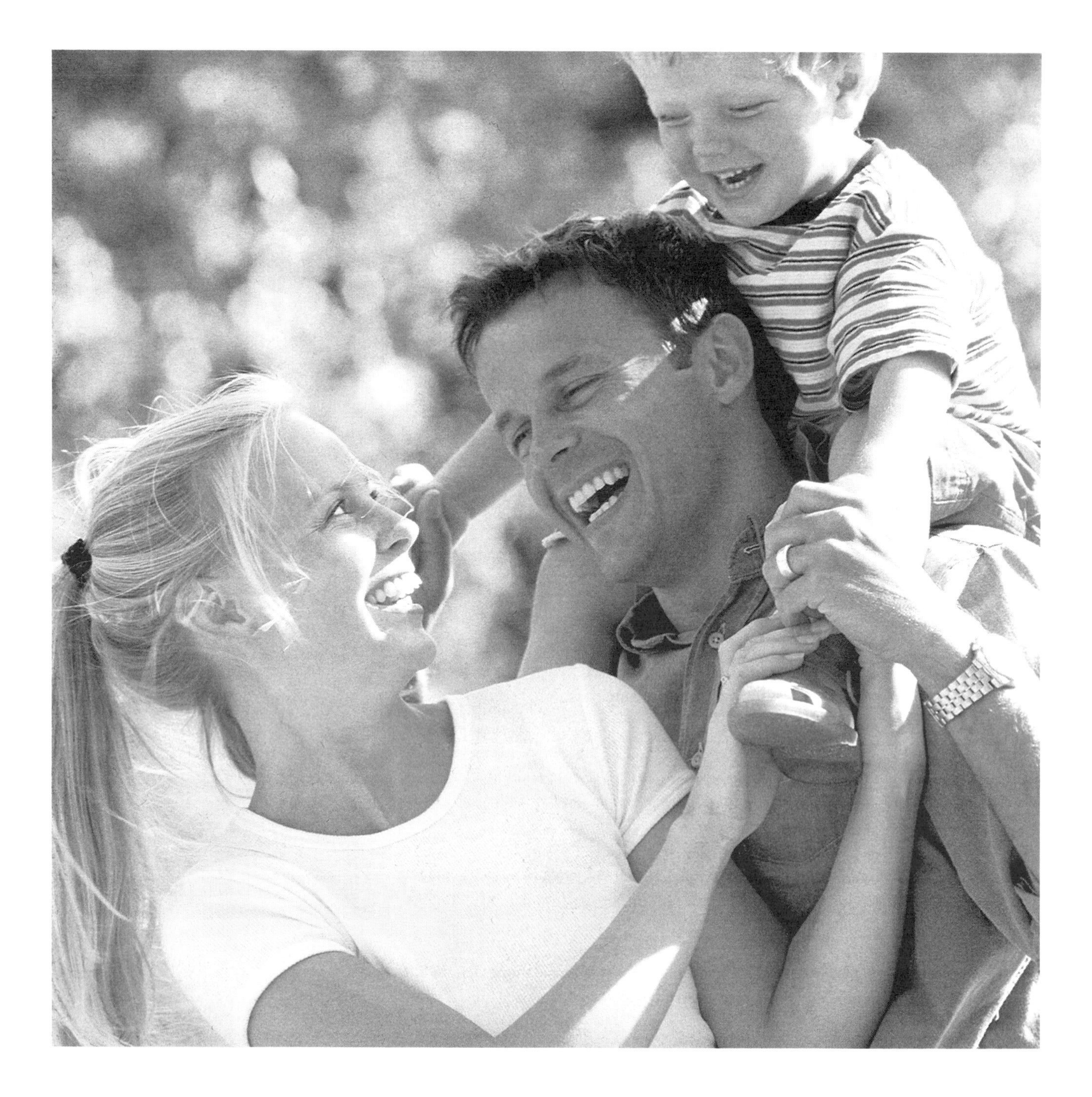

Section Three: The most important Minerals

Boron

WHAT IT IS Boron is a trace element.

WHAT IT DOES Boron interacts with several enzymes and is thought to be important for normal brain function by affecting the movement of chemicals across nerve cells. It plays a role in bone health by improving absorption of dietary calcium (by promoting production of the active form of vitamin D) and stimulates increased production of oestrogen and testosterone hormones.

FOOD SOURCES Foods containing Boron include:

- Fresh fruit, nuts and green vegetables

HOW MUCH YOU NEED A daily intake of 3mg is suggested as optimum for bone health. A safe upper limit of 9.6mg boron per day has been suggested for adults.

DEFICIENCY It has been suggested that osteoporosis is a condition linked with boron-deficiency.

RESEARCH Post-menopausal women taking boron supplements (3mg daily) for 7 weeks lost less calcium and magnesium from their body than when following a low boron diet. Their production of both oestrogen and testosterone hormones also doubled and may help to reduce the risk of osteoporosis.

SIDE EFFECTS/SAFETY Toxicity can occur at intakes of 100mg per day or more. Symptoms of toxicity can include headache, muscle pain, nausea, vomiting, red eyes, rash and peeling skin.

WHAT TO LOOK FOR WHEN SELECTING A SUPPLEMENT

Supplements aimed at the over 50s should ideally include boron.

Calcium

WHAT IT IS Calcium is the most abundant mineral in our body, with 99% (around 1.2kg) found in our bones and teeth in the form of hydroxyapatite. Absorption of calcium in the small intestine depends upon the presence of vitamin D.

WHAT IT DOES Good intakes of calcium are vital throughout life for the growth, development and maintenance of strong, healthy bones and teeth. Calcium also plays a vital role in muscle contraction, nerve conduction, blood clotting, energy production and the regulation of many important metabolic enzymes.

FOOD SOURCES Foods containing Calcium include:

- milk, dairy products such as cheese, yoghurt, fromage frais (but not butter), green leafy vegetables eg broccoli, tinned salmon (including the bones), nuts and seeds, pulses, white and brown bread (in the UK, white and brown flour are fortified with calcium by law - but not wholemeal flour) and eggs

Less than 40% of dietary calcium is absorbed from the gut and lack of calcium is common.

Drinking an extra pint of skimmed or semi-skimmed milk per day provides an additional 720mg calcium in the readily absorbed form of calcium lactate.

- ✖ Processing can reduce the mineral content of foods by up to 80%.
- ✖ Further losses occur by leaching into water during freezing or cooking.
- ✖ Some types of fibre (eg phytates from wheat in unleavened bread) bind calcium in the bowel to form an insoluble, non-absorbable salt.
- ✖ High fibre diets, which speed the passage of food through the bowels, also reduce the amount of calcium absorbed.

HOW MUCH YOU NEED The EC RDA for calcium is 800mg. Some adults may need more – between 1000mg and 1500mg if their risk of osteoporosis is high.

Taking up to1500mg calcium supplements daily appears to be safe, although high doses should usually be taken together with other minerals such as zinc, iron and magnesium whose absorption it also affects.

DEFICIENCY

When dietary calcium is in short supply, it is leached from the body instead to help maintain a healthy heart beat. As a result, bone thinning (osteoporosis) can develop when calcium intakes are low.

Symptoms that may be due to minor lack:

- infected gums (periodontal disease)
- muscle aches and pains
- muscle twitching and spasm
- muscle cramps

Symptoms that may be due to major deficiency:

- tetany (sustained cramps)
- palpitations
- receding gums
- loose teeth
- convulsions
- dementia

RESEARCH Lack of calcium at any stage in life increases the risk of future osteoporosis.

Adding calcium supplements to the diet of elderly people reduces their risk of a vertebral fracture by 20%, while giving them both calcium and vitamin D supplements may reduce their risk of non-vertebral and hip fracture by 30% - 40%.

Low intakes of calcium have been linked with high blood pressure and stroke.

Drugs that affect calcium channels in the body are highly successful in treating hypertension, angina, some irregular heart rhythms and poor circulation.

SIDE EFFECTS/SAFETY Calcium tablets are best taking with meals. Some evidence suggests they are better taken with your evening meal rather than breakfast as calcium flux is greatest in the body at night, when growth hormone is secreted.

People with a tendency towards kidney stones should ideally take calcium supplements together with essential fatty acids but seek medical advice first.

Those taking certain tetracycline antibiotics will need to ensure they do not eat or drink calcium containing foods for at least an hour either side of taking their medication, as calcium binds with some tetracyclines to reduce their absorption.

WHAT TO LOOK FOR WHEN SELECTING A SUPPLEMENT Calcium in the form of calcium lactate, calcium gluconate, calcium malate and calcium citrate are most easily absorbed from the intestines. Calcium citrate is less likely to cause constipation than calcium carbonate, and is also better for older people who may produce less stomach acid).

Taking calcium supplements together with essential fatty acids (eg evening primrose or fish oils) increases the amount of calcium that is absorbed and deposited in bones.

Divide high doses into two or even three daily doses to improve absorption.

Chromium

WHAT IT IS The trivalent form of chromium used in supplements is a trace element usually supplied as either chromium picolinate or chromium polynicotinate.

WHAT IT DOES Chromium combines with vitamin B3 and three amino acids to form an organic complex known as Glucose Tolerance Factor (GTF). This interacts with insulin hormone to help control the way cells take up glucose for energy.

GTF also encourages the production of energy from glucose, especially in muscles, increases protein synthesis and lowers blood fat levels. It may also suppress hunger pangs through a direct action on the brain.

FOOD SOURCES Foods containing Chromium include:

- egg yolk, red meat, cheese, fruit and fruit juice, wholegrains, honey, condiments eg black pepper, thyme and vegetables

The chromium found in brewer's yeast is already in the form of GTF which is more effective than other sources.

Most refined carbohydrates have little chromium content and people eating processed foods will have low intakes.

- ✖ Processing can reduce the mineral content of foods by up to 80%
- ✖ Further losses occur by leaching into water during freezing or cooking.

HOW MUCH YOU NEED There is no agreed RDA, but intakes of 50 - 200 micrograms per day are thought to be both safe and desirable for adults. In general, the more carbohydrate you eat, the more chromium you need.

DEFICIENCY Chromium deficiency is thought to be common as 90% of people are estimated to get less than 50 mcg from their diet, and only around 2% is in the absorbable (trivalent) form. Low levels of chromium have been linked with poor glucose tolerance and increased risk of developing maturity-onset (insulin independent) diabetes and cardiovascular disease.

Symptoms that may be due to minor lack:

- poor glucose tolerance with either raised or lowered blood sugar levels
- poor tolerance of alcohol
- abnormal blood fat levels
- muscle weakness
- irritability

Symptoms that may be due to major deficiency:

- confusion
- depression
- thirst
- decreased sperm count and impaired fertility

RESEARCH When supplements providing 200mcg chromium per day were given to people with diabetes, almost half needed less insulin or blood sugar-lowering tablets. The effects were twice as good in those with non-insulin dependent diabetes than in those with insulin dependent diabetes.

Chromium may reduce the risk of coronary heart disease by lowering harmful low-density lipoprotein (LDL) cholesterol and raising beneficial high density (HDL) cholesterol.

When combined with a sensible diet and regular exercise, chromium supplements may help some people lose weight, especially if they are deficient in chromium.

SIDE EFFECTS/SAFETY Do not exceed the stated dose, which may affect zinc and iron absorption.

WHAT TO LOOK FOR WHEN SELECTING A SUPPLEMENT Yeast derived GTF is ten times more active than that from any other food and special chromium-enriched yeast strains have now been developed.

Supplements are best absorbed when taken with vitamin C.

Copper

WHAT IT IS Copper is a trace element.

WHAT IT DOES Copper is essential in small amounts for healthy liver, brain and muscle function. It is needed for the production of a number of brain chemicals, the skin pigment, melanin and the red blood pigment, haemoglobin. It plays an important role in oxygen transportation, cellular respiration and the synthesis of collagen. It is therefore involved in maintaining healthy bones, cartilage, hair and skin - especially their elasticity.

Copper is essential for the function of a number of enzymes involved in antioxidant protection (eg superoxide dismutase), and also plays an important role in the metabolism of vitamin C. In fact, if vitamin C intakes are good, copper deficiency can quickly occur.

FOOD SOURCES Foods containing Copper include:

- crustaceans eg prawns, shellfish eg oysters, olives, nuts, pulses, wholegrain cereals, green vegetables grown in copper-rich soil

✖ Processing can reduce the mineral content of foods by up to 80%.

✖ Further losses occur by leaching into water during freezing or cooking.

Up to 70% of dietary intake remains unabsorbed because it is bound to other bowel contents. Supplementation is therefore important, especially if the diet is deficient.

Many people with arthritis have low blood levels of copper, and are helped by wearing a copper bracelet so trace amounts are absorbed through the skin.

HOW MUCH YOU NEED There is no EC RDA for copper. Intakes between 0.8mg and 3mg are believed to be both safe and adequate for adults.

DEFICIENCY Lack of copper can occur in some conditions such as Crohn's or coeliac disease or in people with hereditary inability to process copper properly. This can lead to heart muscle problems (cardiac myopathy).

RESEARCH Copper is believed to have a role in regulating blood cholesterol levels and may protect against hardening and furring up of the arteries (atherosclerosis).

Menopausal women taking 3mg copper supplements per day did not lose as much bone density as those taking placebo suggesting that supplements may help to prevent osteoporosis.

SIDE EFFECTS/SAFETY Excess copper (eg from drinking water supplied through copper pipes) is toxic at levels just twice as high as usual can cause restlessness, nausea, vomiting, colic, diarrhoea. Long term high intakes can lead to copper-induced cirrhosis of the liver.

Symptoms that may be due to minor lack:

- increased susceptibility to infection
- loss of taste sensation
- irritability

Symptoms that may be due to major deficiency:

- pallor (anaemia)
- fluid retention
- raised blood cholesterol levels
- abnormal structure and pigmentation of body hair
- abnormal pigmentation and loss of elasticity in skin
- nerve degeneration
- impaired fertility

WHAT TO LOOK FOR WHEN SELECTING A SUPPLEMENT The ideal dietary ratio of copper to zinc is 1:10.

Iodine

WHAT IT IS Iodine is a trace element.

WHAT IT DOES Iodine is essential for the production of two thyroid hormones, thyroxine and tri-iodothyronine. These hormones control the metabolic rate, the conversion of food and fat stores into energy and the production of body heat. Iodine helps to prevent lack of energy, tiredness and excessive weight gain.

FOOD SOURCES Foods containing Iodine include:

- marine fish eg haddock, halibut, salmon, tuna, seafood (eg prawns, mussels, lobster, oysters), seaweed (eg kelp), iodised salt, milk (cattle feed is also iodised), crops and cattle reared on soils exposed to sea-spray

✖ Processing can reduce the mineral content of foods by up to 80%.

✖ Further losses occur by leaching into water during freezing or cooking.

HOW MUCH YOU NEED The EC RDA for iodine is 150 mcg per day Those who are physically active may need more iodine than people who are inactive, as iodine is lost in sweat - an athlete in heavy training can lose the full iodine RDA in sweat alone. Intakes of up to 0.5mg per day are not expected to cause significant side effects.

DEFICIENCY Gross iodine deficiency leading to swelling of the thyroid gland (goitre) is now rare in the UK since the introduction of iodised salt. People who restrict their salt intake and who do not eat iodine-rich foods (eg seafood) are at risk of iodine deficiency however, and in some parts of the world, including parts of Europe, New Zealand, Brazil and the Himalayas, iodine deficiency is relatively common.

Selenium plays a role in the metabolism of thyroid hormones, and the effects of iodine deficiency are made worse by low selenium intakes.

Symptoms that may be due to minor lack:

- tiredness
- lack of energy
- muscle weakness
- breast pain and tenderness
- increased production of mucus

Symptoms that may be due to major deficiency:

- susceptibility to the cold
- thyroid goitre
- brittle, coarse hair
- weight gain
- coarse skin

RESEARCH In the Western world, newborn babies are screened for cretinism which results from lack of iodine as part of the heel prick test carried out soon after delivery.

SIDE EFFECTS/SAFETY Up to 3% of people are allergic to iodine.

Excess iodine may lead to a metallic taste in the mouth, oral sores, headache, diarrhoea, vomiting, rash and – as with a deficiency – can also lead to thyroid swelling (goitre).

WHAT TO LOOK FOR WHEN SELECTING A SUPPLEMENT

Iodine is best obtained from natural extracts of kelp, bladderwrack (Fucus) or from an A to Z type vitamin and mineral supplement.

Iron

WHAT IT IS Iron is an essential metallic mineral.

WHAT IT DOES Iron is needed for production of the red blood pigment, haemoglobin (which transports oxygen and carbon dioxide around the body) and the red muscle pigment, myoglobin (which binds oxygen in muscle cells for ready access during exercise). Many enzyme systems rely on iron, including those involved in the production of energy from carbohydrate, fat and protein and immunity. White blood cells destroy invading micro-organisms using powerful iron-containing chemicals.

FOOD SOURCES Foods containing Iron include:

- red meat, offal (liver, kidney, heart), shellfish, fish, especially sardines, wheatgerm, wholemeal bread, egg yolk, green vegetables and prunes and other dried fruit

The form of iron that is most easily absorbed is organic haem iron found in red meat.

✖ Processing can reduce the mineral content of foods by up to 80%.

✖ Further losses occur by leaching into water during freezing or cooking

✖ Overboiling vegetables decreases their iron availability by up to 20%.

Coffee can reduce iron absorption by up to 39% if drunk within an hour of eating. Vegetarians, and those who eat little red meat are at increased risk of iron deficiency. Their intakes are dependent on absorbing inorganic non-haem iron, and food supplements are essential.

Vitamin C increases the absorption of inorganic iron whilst calcium and tannin-containing drinks (eg tea) decreases it.

HOW MUCH YOU NEED The EC RDA for iron is 14mg for adults. A low upper safe level of 17mg per day has been suggested for guidance purposes. Higher amounts are given to treat iron-deficiency anaemia but these often cause intestinal side effects.

DEFICIENCY Lack of iron leads to the production of red blood cells that are much smaller and paler than normal, leading to iron-deficiency anaemia.

World-wide, iron deficiency is the commonest nutritional disease. Women are most at risk because of blood loss during the menstrual cycle.

Symptoms that may be due to minor lack:

- tiredness
- muscle fatigue
- generalised skin itching
- dizziness
- headache
- insomnia
- decreased appetite
- brittle hair and hair loss

Symptoms that may be due to major deficiency:

- pallor (anaemia)
- concave, brittle nails
- sore tongue
- cracking at the corners of the mouth
- increased susceptibility to infection
- difficulty swallowing

Iron deficiency can cause an increased susceptibility to infection, especially recurrent thrush and Herpes simplex virus infections.

RESEARCH Up to 20% of the menstruating women in developed countries are iron deficient, but less than half of these have anaemia (haemoglobin level less than 12g/dl). Low iron levels are best detected by measuring the amount of iron-binding protein (ferritin) present in the circulation.

While optimum intakes of iron are important, some studies suggest that excess intakes may increase the risk of heart disease and colon cancer, especially in males. Supplements designed for older people (eg over 50s) therefore usually contain less iron than those aimed at younger adults.

SIDE EFFECTS/SAFETY Side effects of nausea, indigestion, constipation and dark-coloured bowel motions are common with higher dose iron supplements. If you think you have anaemia, always seek medical advice before taking iron supplements, as the cause needs to be determined and iron supplements may mask iron deficiency.

Avoid taking too much iron as this can cause constipation or indigestion and excess is toxic (especially for children).

Keep iron supplements away from small children – eating just a few have been known to kill.

What to look for when selecting a supplement

Iron is best taken on an empty stomach unless this causes irritation.

Ferrous fumarate or ferrous gluconate is usually better tolerated than ferrous sulphate.

Iron supplements given alone can decrease the absorption of zinc, and other essential minerals (eg manganese, chromium and selenium) so it is usually advisable to only take iron in combination with these eg in an A to Z type vitamin and mineral supplement (unless prescribed individually by a doctor).

Magnesium

WHAT IT IS Magnesium is an essential mineral. Seventy per cent of body stores are found in the bones and teeth.

WHAT IT DOES Magnesium is important for maintaining the integrity of body cells. Special salt pumps maintain different ion concentration gradients across cell walls that allow them to hold an electrical charge and pass electrical messages from one cell to another. Magnesium is essential for maintaining these membrane pumps and a cell's electrical stability. It is especially important in controlling calcium entry into heart cells to trigger a regular heart beat.

Magnesium is vital for every major metabolic reaction from the synthesis of protein and genetic material to the production of energy from glucose. Few enzymes can work without it.

FOOD SOURCES Foods containing Magnesium include:

- seafood, seaweed, meat, eggs, dairy products, wholegrains, soya beans, nuts, bananas, dark green, leafy vegetables and chocolate

✖ Processing can reduce the mineral content of foods by up to 80%.

✖ Further losses occur by leaching into water during freezing or cooking.

HOW MUCH YOU NEED The EC RDA for magnesium is 300mg. Intakes of up to 400mg per day would not be expected to cause adverse effects.

People who are physically active may need more magnesium, as large amounts can be lost in sweat.

DEFICIENCY Lack of magnesium is common and may affect as many as one in ten people.

Symptoms that may be due to minor lack:

- loss of appetite
- nausea
- fatigue
- weakness
- pre-menstrual syndrome
- insomnia
- diarrhoea

Symptoms that may be due to major deficiency:

- muscle trembling or cramps
- numbness and tingling
- loss of co-ordination
- constipation
- confusion
- nervousness
- palpitations
- dizziness
- difficult or painful swallowing

RESEARCH People with low levels of magnesium are more at risk of spasm of the coronary arteries (linked with angina or heart attack) and spasm of airways leading to asthma.

Magnesium treatment is sometimes given immediately after a heart attack to help prevent dangerous abnormal heart rhythms. It also helps to widen coronary blood vessels, and reduces the formation of platelet blood clots.

As magnesium regulates the movement of calcium in and out of cells, it is important for bone health and preventing osteoporosis.

Low levels have also been linked with chronic fatigue and pre-menstrual syndrome.

SIDE EFFECTS/SAFETY Best taken with food to optimise absorption.

WHAT TO LOOK FOR WHEN SELECTING A SUPPLEMENT Magnesium citrate is most readily absorbed, while magnesium gluconate is less likely to cause intestinal side effects such as diarrhoea at higher doses. When taking magnesium supplements, ensure you also have a good intake of calcium.

WHAT IT IS Manganese is an essential trace element.

WHAT IT DOES Manganese is needed for the synthesis of cartilage, collagen and structural molecules known as mucopolysaccharides. It therefore plays an important role in normal growth and development, especially of bones. It is involved in many metabolic functions, including the synthesis of amino acids, carbohydrates, blood clotting factors, cholesterol and some hormones and brain chemicals. It also acts as an antioxidant.

FOOD SOURCES Foods containing Manganese include:

- Tea (1mg per cup, on average), whole grains, nuts and seeds, fruits, egg, green leafy vegetables/herbs, offal, shellfish and milk

✖ Processing can reduce the mineral content of foods by up to 80%.

✖ Further losses occur by leaching into water during freezing or cooking.

HOW MUCH YOU NEED There is no EC RDA for manganese, but an intake of up to 10mg per day is believed to be both safe and adequate. Some researchers suggest that up to 7mg manganese are needed daily for optimum bone health.

DEFICIENCY Up to 4mg manganese is lost in bowel motions each day, which needs to be replaced. The significance of manganese deficiency is currently unknown.

Symptoms that may be due to minor lack:

- reddening of body hair
- scaly skin
- poor growth of hair and nails
- disc and cartilage problems
- poor memory

Symptoms that may be due to major deficiency:

- impaired blood clotting
- glucose intolerance
- worsening intellect
- middle ear problems
- reduced fertility

RESEARCH Women with osteoporosis have been found to have manganese levels that were four times lower than those without osteoporosis.

SIDE EFFECTS/SAFETY Industrial workers exposed to inhalation of manganese dust have experienced toxicity – known as manganism - with nervous system effects similar to Parkinson's disease.

WHAT IT IS Phosphorus is a mineral that makes up at least half a kilogram of your body weight. Ninety per cent is found in your bones and teeth where it forms calcium phosphate - a hard mineral salt also known as hydroxyapatite.

WHAT IT DOES As well as forming part of the major structural mineral in bones and teeth, phosphorus is also found in muscle cells where it is essential for the production of energy-rich molecules. Phosphorus is also an important component of the chemicals making up our genetic information.

FOOD SOURCES Foods containing Phosphorus include:

- Fish, poultry, meat, dairy products, wholegrain cereals, soya beans, nuts, eggs and yeast extract

Vitamin D is essential for absorption of phosphorus and calcium from the gut and for their deposition in bone.

- ✖ Processing can reduce the mineral content of foods by up to 80%.
- ✖ Further losses occur by leaching into water during freezing or cooking.

HOW MUCH YOU NEED Phosphorus requirements are usually set the same as for calcium. The EC RDA for phosphorus is therefore 800mg.

DEFICIENCY

Deficiency can develop in people using antacids containing aluminium hydroxide long term which impairs absorption of phosphates from the gut.

Symptoms that may be due to minor lack:

- general malaise
- loss of appetite
- increased susceptibility to infection
- anaemia

Symptoms that may be due to major deficiency:

- muscle weakness and tremor
- bone pain
- joint stiffness
- numbness
- pins and needles
- irritability
- confusion

RESEARCH Tests with endurance athletes have found that taking phosphate supplements for three days before a competition decreases lactic acid build up in muscles, increases oxygen consumption and stamina, as well as increasing maximal power output.

SIDE EFFECTS/SAFETY High intakes can cause diarrhoea.

WHAT TO LOOK FOR WHEN SELECTING A SUPPLEMENT Few people are at risk of phosphorus deficiency, and single supplements are rarely needed. Low doses are included in some vitamin and mineral products for completeness.

Phosphorus should be given together with calcium to prevent abnormal calcium metabolism in the body.

Potassium

WHAT IT IS Potassium is a mineral that is mainly found inside body cells.

WHAT IT DOES Cells accumulate potassium by swapping it for sodium via the so-called sodium potassium pumps found in all cell membranes. Potassium is essential for normal muscle contraction, generation of a regular heart beat, conduction of messages along nerve fibres, and for the maintenance of blood sugar levels. It is also involved in the production of genetic material, proteins and energy. The kidney regulates blood potassium levels and keeps them within a fairly narrow range.

FOOD SOURCES Foods containing Potassium include:

- seafood, fruit, vegetables, wholegrains, rock salt and 'low sodium' salts
- ✖ Processing can reduce the mineral content of foods by up to 80%.
- ✖ Further losses occur by leaching into water during freezing or cooking.

HOW MUCH YOU NEED There is no EC RDA for potassium but intakes of around 3000mg to 3500mg daily are thought to be both safe and adequate.

DEFICIENCY People taking some types of diuretic drugs to reduce water retention may lose potassium through their kidneys and become deficient.

Symptoms that may be due to minor lack:

- poor appetite
- fatigue
- weakness
- muscle cramps
- constipation

Symptoms that may be due to major deficiency:

- irregular or rapid heart beat
- vomiting
- irritability
- headache
- depression
- tissue swelling
- pins and needles
- low blood pressure
- low blood sugar
- bone, joint and muscle pain
- mental confusion
- drowsiness

RESEARCH Diets that are relatively high in potassium and low in sodium are linked with a lower risk of high blood pressure and stroke.

In one study, over 80% of people taking anti-hypertensive medication were able to halve their dose of drug (under medical supervision) just by increasing the potassium content of their food.

SIDE EFFECTS/SAFETY If you have kidney problems, are taking diuretics or a type of medication called an ACE inhibitor, seek medical advice before taking a supplement containing potassium.

The body usually maintains potassium levels within tight limits. High levels can cause irregular heart beat, and muscle fatigue. Very high levels can have dangerous effects on heart rhythm.

WHAT TO LOOK FOR WHEN SELECTING A SUPPLEMENT If phosphate is present, the amount supplied is usually similar to the amount of calcium provided.

Selenium

WHAT IT IS Selenium is an essential trace element.

WHAT IT DOES Selenium is essential for cell growth and immune function. It is involved in the synthesis of hormone-like substances known as prostaglandins and thyroid hormones. Because of its antioxidant action, selenium protects against a wide variety of degenerative diseases such as hardening and furring up of the arteries, emphysema, liver problems, cataracts, arthritis, stroke, heart attack and possibly even cancer. Selenium is also important for immunity, stimulating the production of natural killer cells which fight viral and bacterial infections as well as being involved in the production of antibodies.

FOOD SOURCES Foods containing Selenium include:

- Brazil nuts – the richest dietary source, seafood, offal, wholegrains, onions, garlic, broccoli, cabbage, mushrooms, radishes and celery

The selenium content of vegetables depends on the soils in which they are grown.

✖ Processing can reduce the mineral content of foods by up to 80%.

✖ Further losses occur by leaching into water during freezing or cooking.

HOW MUCH YOU NEED There is no EC RDA for selenium, but intakes of around 75mcg have been suggested. Supplements supplying 100mcg to 200mcg have significant protective effects against cancer.

An upper safe level of 300mcg daily has recently been suggested.

DEFICIENCY A healthy diet can no longer provide adequate intakes of selenium in many parts of Europe. Between 1975 and 1994, selenium intakes almost halved in the UK from 60mcg to 34 mcg per day.

In parts of the world where soil selenium levels are low, the incidence of cancer increases. These risks seem to be even higher if intakes of vitamin E and vitamin A are also low. In parts of China, selenium intakes are low enough to cause a form of heart failure known as Keshan Disease and a form of muscle and joint degeneration known as Kashin-Beck disease.

Symptoms that may be due to minor lack:

- hair, nail and skin problems
- age spots
- premature wrinkling of skin
- poor growth
- subfertility

Symptoms that may be due to major deficiency:

- thyroid problems
- arthritis
- high blood pressure
- cataracts
- some cancers
- muscle weakness
- Keshan disease (a form of heart failure)

RESEARCH Research suggests antibody synthesis increases up to thirty fold if supplements of selenium and vitamin E - which work together as powerful antioxidants - are taken.

In a study involving over 1300 people, those receiving 200mcg selenium a day had a 52% lower risk of cancer death compared with those receiving placebo.

A study looking at the effects of 200mcg selenium supplementation in people with previous skin cancer found significant reductions in total cancer deaths. The trial was therefore stopped early as it was considered unethical to withhold selenium from those in the placebo groups.

Selenium levels are around 10% lower in people with chronic inflammatory conditions such as rheumatoid arthritis.

Low selenium levels seem to increase the risk of miscarriage.

SIDE EFFECTS/SAFETY Toxicity can occur with intakes above 800mcg daily, leading to a garlic odour on the breath, fragile or black fingernails, a metallic taste in the mouth, dizziness, nausea and hair loss.

WHAT TO LOOK FOR WHEN SELECTING A SUPPLEMENT Supplements in which selenium is organically bound to yeast may be more readily absorbed and usable than inorganic selenium salts.

Zinc

WHAT IT IS Zinc is an essential trace element.

WHAT IT DOES Zinc is essential for the proper function of over a hundred different enzymes. It helps to regulate gene activation and the synthesis of specific proteins in response to hormone triggers. It is vital for growth, sexual maturity, wound healing and immune function.

FOOD SOURCES Foods containing Zinc include:

- red meat, seafood, especially oysters, offal, brewer's yeast, whole grains, pulses, eggs and cheese

✖ Processing can reduce the mineral content of foods by up to 80%.

✖ Further losses occur by leaching into water during freezing or cooking.

HOW MUCH YOU NEED The EC RDA for zinc is 15mg per day. A safe upper limit of 25mg per day has been suggested for long term use.

DEFICIENCY Many people only obtain half the zinc RDA from their diet and zinc deficiency becomes increasingly common with age. Males are at particular risk, as each time they make love, they lose around 5mg zinc - one third of their daily requirement.

One of the earliest symptoms of zinc deficiency is loss of taste sensation.

RESEARCH Zinc supplements help to reduce the severity of colds and sore throats.

Lack of zinc is associated with an increased risk of prostatitis (inflammation of the prostate gland) in males.

Women with osteoporosis may have lower zinc levels than women with healthy bones.

Zinc supplements may stimulate appetite and improve food intake in people with anorexia nervosa.

Some people with tinnitus have low levels of zinc, in which case supplements help to improve symptoms.

SIDE EFFECTS/SAFETY Zinc toxicity can cause abdominal pain, nausea, vomiting, lethargy, anaemia and dizziness. Zinc affects iron and copper uptake when taken at doses greater than 50mg/day.

Do not take more than 30mg daily long term except under supervision from a qualified nutritionist or doctor.

WHAT TO LOOK FOR WHEN SELECTING A SUPPLEMENT Usually combined with copper.

Symptoms that may be due to minor lack:

- impaired taste sensation
- poor appetite
- increased susceptibility to infection
- cravings for odd foods
- sleep disturbances
- poor hair growth and hair loss
- poor nail growth
- poor growth
- poor wound healing
- skin problems such as eczema, psoriasis, acne
- visual impairment in later life

Symptoms that may be due to major deficiency:

- delayed puberty
- underdeveloped male sex organs
- low sperm count
- impaired fertility
- impotence
- diarrhoea
- visual disturbances
- mental slowing

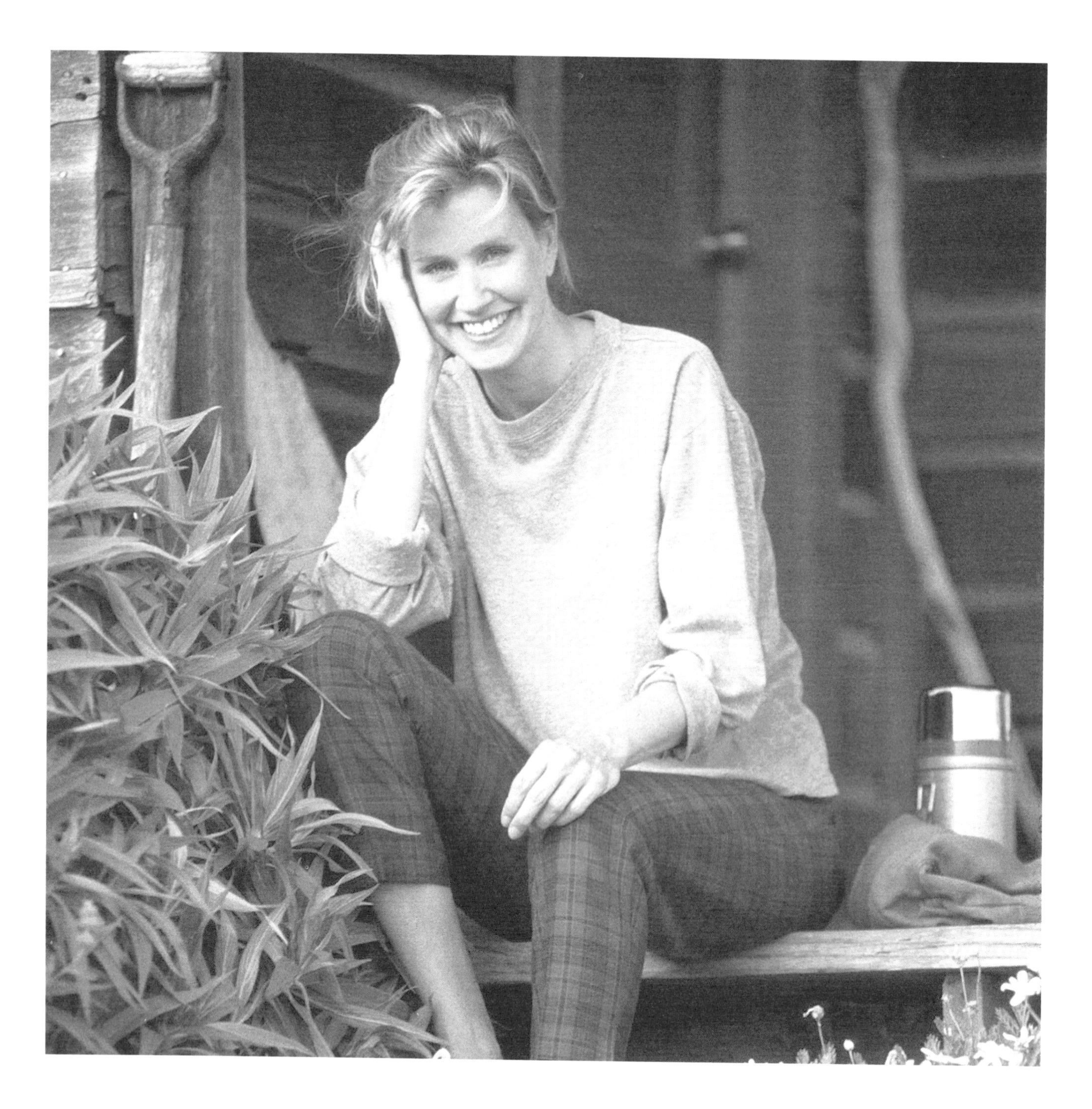

Section Four: The most important Oils

Conjugated Linoleic Acid

WHAT IT IS Conjugated linoleic acid (CLA) is a fatty acid

WHAT IT DOES CLA is involved in cell growth. It has beneficial effects on inflammation, the circulation and blood clotting that can reduce the risk of high blood pressure, high cholesterol levels, heart attack and stroke. It helps to promote the break down of fatty tissue and increase the formation of lean muscle, by interfering with the action of an enzyme (lipoprotein lipase) and by enhancing the body's ability to break down fat stores for energy. CLA may be beneficial for slimmers when combined with a healthy diet and moderate exercise.

HOW MUCH YOU NEED The average diet supplies 100mg to 300mg CLA daily.

The most beneficial intake is thought to be 2000mg daily.

FOOD SOURCES Foods containing CLA include:

- Meat, Dairy products

CLA can also be produced commercially from sunflower, safflower and other oils.

CLA cannot be synthesised in the human body and intakes have fallen due to reduced consumption of meat and dairy products.

RESEARCH Some researchers have claimed that obesity is a CLA deficiency disease, as it is essential for the mobilisation and transport of dietary fats away from fatty tissues to muscle cells where it is burned for fuel. Research has confirmed that CLA helps to reduce the size of fat cells. It seems to help reduce loss of fat around the waist.

CLA may help to reduce regain of fat in people who have successfully lost weight. It may be most effective as a weight management aid rather than a weight loss aid.

It may help to improve glucose control in people with diabetes.

It may help to increase muscle bulk and strength in body builders.

CLA may help to protect against coronary heart disease by reducing blood fat levels and discouraging hardening and furring up of the arteries.

SIDE EFFECTS/SAFETY Do not take during pregnancy as its effects are unknown.

WHAT TO LOOK FOR WHEN SELECTING A SUPPLEMENT Products with a strength of at least 75% CLA are most beneficial. Best taken together with antioxidants to help protect it from oxidation.

Evening Primrose, Starflower & Blackcurrant seed oils

WHAT THEY ARE Evening primrose oil (EPO) is an oil derived from the seed of the Evening primrose plant. EPO is a rich source of gammalinolenic acid (GLA).

A similar oil is extracted from borage (star flower) seeds and from blackcurrant seeds. These oils have a higher content of GLA than evening primrose oil, but also contain other fatty acids that may reduce the amount of GLA absorbed from them.

WHAT THEY DO GLA is processed in the body to form hormone-like substances known as prostaglandins. These help to maintain a healthy hormone balance, and have a beneficial action on inflammation, blood clotting and immunity. It is widely taken to help maintain soft, supple, non-itchy skin and to help improve hormone imbalances associated with breast pain and premenstrual syndrome. It is helpful for people with skin problems such as eczema or psoriasis.

HOW MUCH YOU NEED 1000mg EPO daily for general health (equivalent to 80mg GLA). Up to 3g daily (equivalent to 240mg GLA) may be taken to treat hormone imbalances.

1000mg starflower (borage) oil is equivalent to 3000mg evening primrose oil or 1500mg blackcurrant seed oil.

RESEARCH EPO helps to reduce itching and scaliness in people with eczema.

When taken together with fish oil, people with rheumatoid arthritis were able to reduce their dose of painkillers within six months.

EPO seems to have a beneficial effect on the male prostate gland, reducing symptoms such as urinary frequency.

SIDE EFFECTS/SAFETY The only people who should not take EPO are those who are allergic to it and those with a particular nervous disorder known as temporal lobe epilepsy.

What to look for when selecting a supplement

As an oil, it is best taken with food to boost absorption. It can take up to 3 months to notice a beneficial effect.

WHAT THEY ARE Omega-3 fish oils are extracted from the flesh of oily fish. They are rich in essential fatty acids (EFAs) such as docosahexaenoic acid (DHA) and eicosapentanoic acid (EPA) which are derived from the microalgae on which the fish feed.

Cod liver oil is derived only from the liver of cod. It naturally contains around three times less omega-3 essential fatty acids than is found in oily fish products, but can now be concentrated during processing to increase their percentage. Cod liver oil also contains high amounts of vitamin A and vitamin D.

WHAT THEY DO Omega-3 fish oils help to balance the action of omega-6 oils that are mostly derived from vegetable sources. They have a powerful inflammatory action and are helpful for treating diseases such as asthma, rheumatoid arthritis and psoriasis.

Cod liver oil contains similar omega-3 essential fatty acids as those derived from oily fish and therefore has similar benefits. Usually, however, the only advantage of taking cod liver oil is that it contains fat soluble vitamins, especially vitamins A and D, which have an additional beneficial effect on bones. It is therefore mainly taken for joint problems such as arthritis, but can also benefit the heart and circulation.

HOW MUCH YOU NEED General health 200mg minimum per day.

For optimum benefit, usually 500mg to 4g daily. For severe inflammatory disease, up to 6g daily may be recommended. A good high strength pure omega-3 fish oil formula will provide around 60mg DHA and 90mg EPA per 500mg. A concentrated capsule will provide around 130mg DHA and 200mg EPA per 650mg capsule.

Cod liver oil is usually given in lower doses because of its high vitamin A content. A good quality concentrated cod liver oil capsule may provide 70mg DHA and 50mg EPA per 570mg capsule.

FOOD SOURCES Foods containing Omega-3 Fish Oils include:

- Oily fish (mackerel, herring, salmon, trout, sardines, pilchards)

COD LIVER There is concern that many fish are contaminated with pollutants such as heavy metals, dioxins and PCBs. Some guidelines therefore suggest eating no more than one serving of oily fish per week, whereas two to three servings is ideal. Supplements tested to provide low levels of pollutants may therefore be desirable in place of eating fresh fish! See below.

RESEARCH Omega-3 fish oils can reduce pain, inflammation and swelling in osteoarthritis and rheumatoid arthritis. When evening primrose oil and fish oil were taken in a ratio of 4:1 for six months, nearly all those with rheumatoid arthritis were able to reduce their dose of anti-inflammatory painkilling drugs in one study.

Omega-3 fish oils have a beneficial effect on blood stickiness. In those who have had a heart attack, omega-3 fish oils significantly reduce the chance of a second heart attack. If one does occur, the chances of dying from this second heart attack is significantly decreased. A good intake of oily fish also seems to reduce the risk of dying from a stroke.

Fish oils can reduce the risk of the inflammatory skin disease, psoriasis, by up to 50%. In a study of 80 people with psoriasis, omega-3 fish oils significantly reduced psoriasis patches within 4 to 8 weeks.

A four month study involving people with ulcerative colitis showed that taking fish oil supplements resulted in weight gain and decreased colonic inflammation to the extent that those requiring oral steroids could half drug intakes. In those with Crohn's disease of the bowel, more than two out of three people taking fish oil supplements experienced remission.

OMEGA-3 FISH OIL SUPPLEMENTS CAN IMPROVE PAINFUL PERIODS IN TEENAGE GIRLS. Many fish oil supplements especially designed for pregnancy are now available to help improve development of a baby's eyes and brain, and to help ensure optimum birth weight.

SIDE EFFECTS/SAFETY A recent analysis of marine pollutants such as dioxin and polychlorinated biphenyls (PCBs) in fish oils products carried out by the Food Standards Agency found the lowest levels in products from Guernsey-based Healthspan and from Seven Seas.

Fish oil supplements can cause belching, mild nausea. Shaking fish oil together with milk or juice will emulsify it – break it down into tiny suspended globules that will aid absorption. This is the process that naturally occurs in the stomach and helps to avoid 'fishy burps'. Emulsified fish oil supplements are now widely available, but there is no reason why you shouldn't shake up your own if you find it more pleasant to take.

Do not take cod liver oil products during pregnancy as this contains vitamin A, excess of which can be harmful to a developing baby.

They may worsen asthma in patients who are sensitive to aspirin.

Some research suggests fish oils increase blood sugar levels in diabetics, so monitor sugar levels carefully.

Seek medical advice before taking fish oil supplements if you have a blood clotting disorder or are taking a blood thinning drug such as warfarin (may increase tendency to bleed).

Some people are allergic to fish products.

WHAT TO LOOK FOR WHEN SELECTING A SUPPLEMENT Products described as high or extra high strength provide the highest amount of omega-3 fatty acids.

If taking cod liver oil plus a multivitamin, check the total amounts of vitamin A and D you are taking do not exceed recommended doses. Vitamin A is best limited to less than 5,000iu (1,500 mcg) per day although intakes of up to 10,000iu (3,000 mcg) are considered safe. The EC RDA for vitamin D is 5 mcg (200iu) for but those over the age of 50 need double this amount (10mcg = 400iu) as blood levels fall with increasing age.

If pregnant, only select a fish oil supplement especially designed for use during pregnancy and breast feeding.

Emulsified oils help to prevent the fish after-taste that some people find off-putting.

Vitamin E protects fish oils from rancidity.

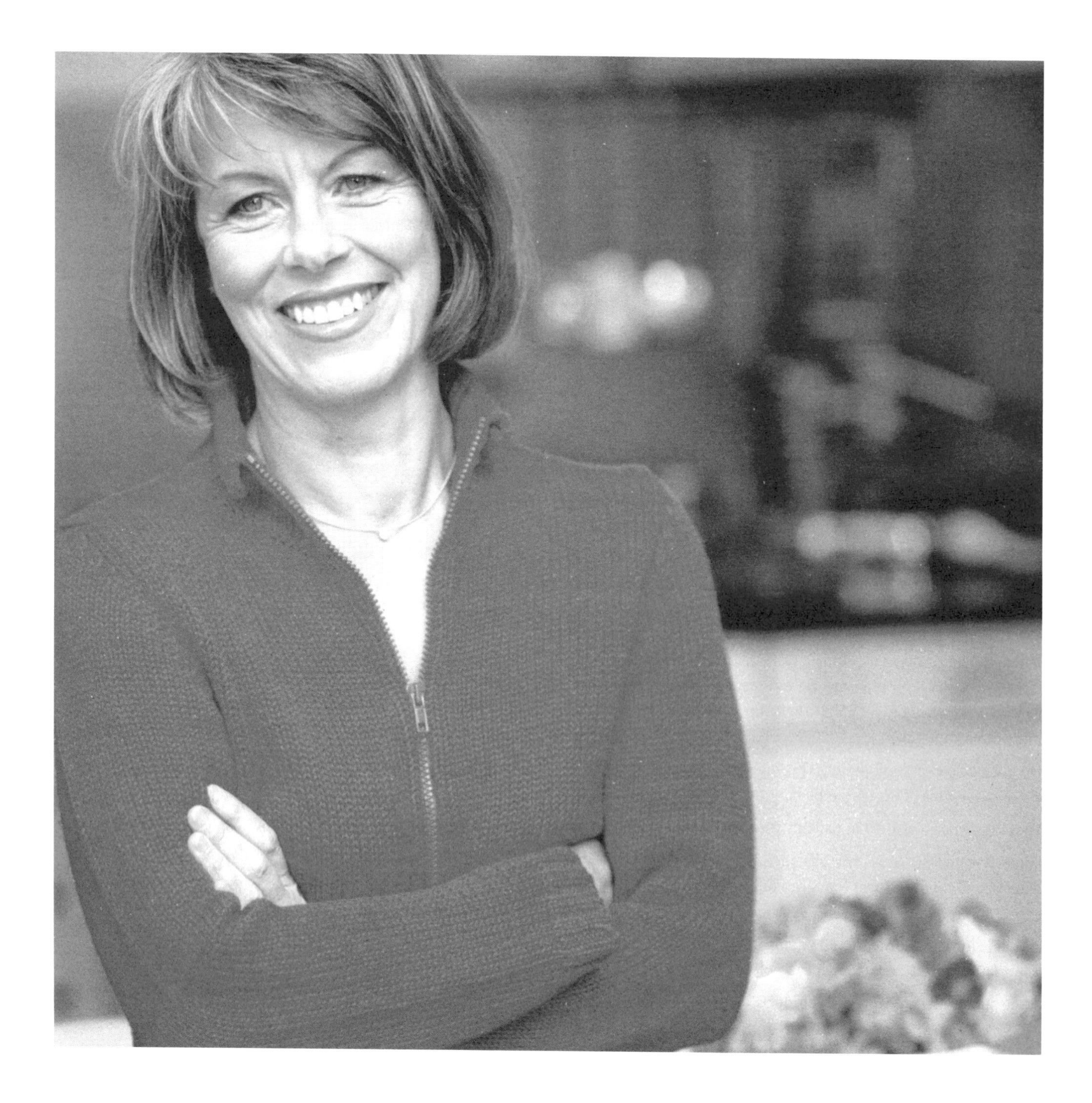

Section Five: The most important Herbal supplements

Agnus castus

WHAT IT IS Agnus castus (Vitex agnus castus) is derived from the fruit of a tree native to the Mediterranean and W. Asia.

WHAT IT DOES Agnus castus is used to help increase sex drive in women, although it has the opposite effect in males. Agnus castus also has a progesterone-like action in women and is valuable in treating pre-menstrual syndrome, polycystic ovary syndrome and menopausal hot flushes. It helps to regularise the menstrual cycle by tending to shorten a long cycle and lengthen a short one. It is also used to help boost female fertility where difficulty in conceiving is thought to be linked with low progesterone levels. Traditionally Agnus castus was used to promote breast milk flow. It has also been used in men to treat male impotence, premature ejaculation, prostatitis, and lack of sexual sensations.

HOW MUCH YOU NEED Extracts standardised to contain 0.5% agnuside: 175 to 225mg daily. Agnus castus is relatively slow acting and may take up to six months to achieve its full effect.

RESEARCH A study of 170 women with PMS found it produced over 50% improvement in symptoms. Greatest improvements were seen in reduction of irritability, mood alteration, anger, headache and breast fullness. Other studies have found it was effective in relieving psychological changes such as increased appetite, sweet cravings, nervousness/ restlessness, anxiety, depression, mood swings and lack of concentration in as many as 90% of cases.

In a study of 45 women with difficulty conceiving due to low progesterone levels, seven became pregnant during the 3 month trial using Agnus castus, and 25 women had their low progesterone levels restored to normal.

SIDE EFFECTS/SAFETY Should be stopped immediately if pregnancy occurs. Should not be taken at the same time as hormone treatments, such as HRT and the oral contraceptive Pill.

Agnus castus should only be used in males under supervision from a qualified medical herbalist. Excess can cause a crawling sensation on the skin known as formication (like ants).

WHAT TO LOOK FOR WHEN SELECTING A SUPPLEMENT Select one standardised to a known amount of agnuside.

Aloe vera

WHAT IT IS Aloe vera is a succulent plant native to Africa. Only three or four out of over 200 different species are used medicinally, the most useful being Aloe vera Barbadensis.

WHAT IT DOES The gel has soothing, anti-inflammatory properties and has been used externally to help treat sunburn, insect bites, eczema, psoriasis, acne, shingles, gum disease, to hasten wound healing and as a cleansing antiseptic against bacterial and fungal infections. Used internally, it is a popular remedy for intestinal disorders such as irritable bowel syndrome, indigestion, constipation, diverticulosis, ulcerative colitis and Crohn's disease. It is also believed to have immune-stimulating properties.

HOW MUCH YOU NEED Aloe latex: one teaspoon to 2 tablespoons daily for a laxative effect.

Aloe very juice: 50 to 100ml three times daily. Super strength tablets: 1000mg – 2000mg daily.

RESEARCH An ointment containing aloe vera gel, applied three times a day, healed over 80% of psoriasis plaques within four weeks compared with only 8% with placebo.

SIDE EFFECTS/SAFETY Avoid during pregnancy, as there is some suggesting that it may stimulate uterine contractions to increase the risk of miscarriage.

Avoid during breast-feeding.

It should not be applied to infected deep (eg surgical) wounds however as some evidence suggests it may increase the time taken for wounds to heal.

Some Aloe vera products contain the bitter aloe 'latex' extracted from the inner yellow leaves of the plant. This will produce a brisk laxative response within 8 to 12 hours.

Some women using Aloe vera notice that it increases their menstrual flow.

WHAT TO LOOK FOR WHEN SELECTING A SUPPLEMENT When selecting a product, aim for one made from 100% pure aloe vera. Its strength needs to be at least 40% by volume to be effective and ideally approaching 95% to 100%.

Select a product that is aloin-free unless you want the laxative effect.

Artichoke

WHAT IT IS Globe artichoke (Cynara scolymus)is a plant native to the Mediterranean. Its leaves contain several unique substances such as cynarin.

WHAT IT DOES Globe artichoke helps to increase bile secretion and improve digestion of dietary fats. This helps to improve digestive symptoms such as bloating, flatulence, nausea and abdominal pain due to intestinal spasm. It has a similar action to milk thistle in protecting liver cells from the ill effects of toxins – especially alcohol – and is also known to help reduce cholesterol levels and protect against hardening and furring up of the arteries. Artichoke extracts also have a mild diuretic action and act as an antioxidant.

HOW MUCH YOU NEED 320mg – 360mg capsules, one to six daily, with food. Concentrated extracts can supply the equivalent of as much as 9000mg fresh globe artichoke leaves per 360mg tablet (25:1).

RESEARCH Taking 320mg artichoke extracts was shown to increase bile secretion by over 127% after 30 minutes, rising to 151% after 60 minutes.

A study involving 279 people with symptoms of irritable bowel syndrome found that standardised artichoke supplements reduced symptoms by 71% within an average of 10 days. One in three noticed an improvement within one week.

A study involving over 550 people showed that taking artichoke extracts for six weeks reduced nausea, vomiting, abdominal pain and constipation by at least 70%.

Artichoke leaf extracts were shown to lower cholesterol levels by 11.5% and triglyceride levels by 12.5%.

SIDE EFFECTS/SAFETY Do not use if you have known obstruction of bile ducts. If you have gallstones, use only after medical advice.

Do not take during pregnancy or breast-feeding unless advised to by a doctor or medical herbalist.

WHAT TO LOOK FOR WHEN SELECTING A SUPPLEMENT Select a standardised product containing a known amount of cynarin eg 7.2mg.

Black Cohosh

WHAT IT IS Black Cohosh (Cimicifuga racemosa) is a Canadian herb also known as Squaw root or black snakeroot. Its root contains hormone-like substances such as formononetin.

WHAT IT DOES Black Cohosh is an adaptogen that helps to balance female hormones. It is mainly used to help relieve menopausal hot flushes and night sweats, but is also used to help relax menstrual cramps, treat painful or irregular periods, low libido, hormone imbalances and pre-menstrual syndrome. It is especially helpful in reducing feelings of depression, anxiety, tension, and mood swings. Black Cohosh is thought to decrease ovarian output of progesterone hormone to normalise oestrogen-progesterone balance. It also has a direct action on centres of the brain that help to control dilation of blood vessels, to reduce menopausal symptoms of hot flushes and sweating.

HOW MUCH YOU NEED 10mg to 160mg standardised extracts daily.

RESEARCH Standardised extracts of Black Cohosh are at least as effective as prescribed HRT in relieving hot flushes, vaginal dryness, depression and anxiety. In another study, Black Cohosh out performed diazepam and oestrogen HRT in relieving depressive moods and anxiety. Four out of five women taking it describe its effects as either good or very good.

Black Cohosh plus St John's Wort was effective in treating 78% of women with hot flushes and other menopausal problems.

SIDE EFFECTS/SAFETY No serious side effects have been reported. Excess may cause headache, nausea or indigestion.

Black Cohosh should not be taken during pregnancy or when breast-feeding.

Because its unique oestrogen action does not stimulate oestrogen-sensitive tumours (and may even inhibit them) Black Cohosh extracts have been used in women with a history of breast cancer although this should only be done under the supervision of a qualified herbalist.

WHAT TO LOOK FOR WHEN SELECTING A SUPPLEMENT Select a standardised product supplying a known amount of triterpene glycosides (eg 2.5%).

Cranberry

WHAT IT IS Cranberries (Vaccinium macrocarpon) are red berries from a shrub native to N. America.

WHAT IT DOES Cranberry juice is drunk for its high vitamin C content, and for its beneficial effect in reducing the incidence of urinary infections. Cranberries contain a type of chemical (anti-adhesin) that prevents bacteria sticking to cells lining the urinary tract wall, so they are more easily flushed out. Drinking 300ml cranberry juice daily (25% strength) can almost halve the risk of developing cystitis. Cranberry is also helpful for reducing the unpleasant odours associated with urinary incontinence.

HOW MUCH YOU NEED Cranberry juice: 300ml daily for treatment (200ml for prevention)

Cranberry extracts: 400mg to 800mg daily

RESEARCH When 153 elderly women drank either 300 ml cranberry juice or inactive placebo for six months, those drinking cranberry juice were 42% less likely to develop signs of a urinary infection than those not drinking it. And if signs of infection did develop, the chance of it still being there one month later was only 27% of the odds in those not drinking cranberry juice.

In another trial, 24 women with a history of recurring urinary infections where given antibiotics for six months. Half then continued with antibiotics for the next six months while the other half took just cranberry extracts instead. Among those taking cranberry extracts, only one person developed a urinary tract infection during this time compared with 25 relapses (average of 2.3 per patient) in those continuing with the antibiotics!

SIDE EFFECTS/SAFETY If you think you have a urinary infection, always seek medical advice – especially during pregnancy.

Devil's claw

WHAT IT IS Devil's claw (Harpagophytum procumbens) is a South African desert plant whose tubers contain unique compounds such as harpagoside.

WHAT IT DOES Devil's Claw has a natural, anti-inflammatory, pain-killing action and is taken to treat back or joint pain due to osteoarthritis, rheumatoid arthritis, gout and sport's injuries. Traditionally, it was used as a tonic to aid digestive problems, headaches and to reduce fevers. It also encourages excretion of uric acid to reduce the risk of recurrent gout.

HOW MUCH YOU NEED 1g to 10g daily depending on concentration

A typical 440mg tablet standardised extract is equivalent to 2200mg powdered root.

RESEARCH A double-blind, placebo-controlled trial showed significant reductions in muscle pain, pain sensitivity and muscle tension in those suffering from shoulder neck and back pain with benefits appearing after around two weeks of treatment.

SIDE EFFECTS/SAFETY Take with food. Do not take if you have peptic ulcers or indigestion as it promotes secretion of digestive juices.

Avoid during pregnancy and breastfeeding.

WHAT TO LOOK FOR WHEN SELECTING A SUPPLEMENT Look for a supplement standardised to a known amount of harpagoside eg minimum of 1.5% providing 6mg per tablet.

Take for a minimum of four weeks to achieve maximum effect.

Echinacea

WHAT IT IS Echinacea is a traditional Native American Indian remedy derived from the flowers and leaves of the Purple Coneflower (Echinacea purpurea). Echinacea contains several unique substances known as echinacins.

WHAT IT DOES Echinacea helps to stimulate the immune system. It increases the number and activity of white blood cells so they are more likely to absorb and destroy viral, fungal and bacterial infections. It also seems to boost production of the body's own natural anti-viral substance called interferon. It also contains flavonoids that have an antioxidant action.

Echinacea helps to prevent and treat recurrent upper respiratory tract infections such as the common cold, laryngitis, tonsillitis, otitis media, sinusitis, acne and Herpes cold sores.

HOW MUCH YOU NEED 300mg three times daily to treat colds and 'flu, 200mg three or four times a day for lesser infections

May be used low dose, long term, to reduce infections, or in high dose just when you feel an infection coming on. Concentrated tablets can provide the equivalent of as much as 3200mg fresh herb per 160mg (20:1).

RESEARCH Most studies show Echinacea reduces susceptibility to colds by around a third. On average, it seems to lengthen time between infections by around 60%.

SIDE EFFECTS/SAFETY Some manufacturers prefer their products to be used intermittently eg for no more than two weeks without a break. Always follow manufacturer's guidelines, as different products contain a different balance of ingredients.

No serious side effects have been reported, and it seems to be safe during pregnancy and breastfeeding, although as with all supplements it should only be taken during pregnancy under supervision from a qualified practitioner.

WHAT TO LOOK FOR WHEN SELECTING A SUPPLEMENT Select products standardised to contain at least 3.5% echinicosides, or 3% cichoric acid.

Garlic

WHAT IT IS Garlic (Allium sativum) is a popular kitchen herb. The main beneficial substance derived from garlic is allicin, which gives a crushed clove its characteristic smell. Allicin is present in whole garlic cloves as an odourless precursor called alliin. When garlic is crushed or sliced, alliin comes into contact with a garlic enzyme, alliinase, which breaks it down into the powerful smelling, beneficial allicin.

WHAT IT DOES Garlic has antioxidant, antiseptic, antibacterial and antiviral properties. While it is used to help treat intestinal, respiratory and skin infections, its most important use is to help maintain a healthy heart and circulation. Garlic can reduce high blood pressure, lower levels of harmful blood fats (LDL-cholesterol and triglycerides), reduce blood stickiness, dilate blood vessels and improve blood flow to the peripheries.

HOW MUCH YOU NEED 600mg to 900mg daily. Concentrated capsules are available in which 4mg is equivalent to 800mg fresh garlic bulb. Odour controlled tablets can provide the equivalent of 1200mg fresh garlic bulb, with an allicin yield as high as 2000mcg.

RESEARCH

Allicin lowers cholesterol levels and helps to discourage hardening and furring up of the arteries. Regular use can reduce the risk of hardening and furring up of the arteries up to a quarter.

Garlic extracts have been shown to reduce systolic BP by an average of 8%, reduce the risk of a stroke by up to 40%, and the risk of a heart attack by up to 50% by lowering blood pressure, increasing the fluidity of blood and by helping to maintain the elasticity of important blood vessels. The effects on blood vessel dilation can be seen within 5 hours of taking a single dose, and wear off over 24 hours.

Garlic can improve blood flow to the skin and nail folds by around 50%, and is often used to help improve symptoms of Raynaud's disease and chilblains.

Taking garlic extracts can increase the distance that can be walked for people with calf pain on exercise due to poor circulation.

SIDE EFFECTS/SAFETY Enteric coating of garlic powder tablets reduces garlic odour on breath and protects the active ingredients from degradation in the stomach.

WHAT TO LOOK FOR WHEN SELECTING A SUPPLEMENT Select a product supplying a standardised amount of allicin eg 1500mcg or greater) for heart benefits.

Ginger

WHAT IT IS Ginger (Zingiber officinale) is one of the oldest medicinal spices known. Is derived from the rhizome of a tropical plant native to the jungles of South-east Asia, which contains unique substances such as gingerol and zingerone.

WHAT IT DOES Ginger is used as a warming analgesic, with anti-inflammatory and anti-sickness properties. It is taken to help treat motion and morning sickness, indigestion, flatulence, poor circulation, chilblains, Raynaud's syndrome, colds and fevers. It is also used to help treat muscle and joint aches and pains, including those of rheumatoid and osteoarthritis.

HOW MUCH YOU NEED 100mg to 250mg two to four times daily. A highly concentrated extract may contain 100mg equivalent to 12g powdered ginger root (120:1).

For motion sickness: take three hours before departure.

RESEARCH Gingerol is effective in reducing blood clotting, boosting the circulation and lowering blood pressure.

In a trial involving 247 people with moderate osteoarthritis of the knee, those taking ginger extracts had significantly more pain relief on standing than those taking placebo.

SIDE EFFECTS/SAFETY No serious side effects. Do not exceed recommended doses during pregnancy.

WHAT TO LOOK FOR WHEN SELECTING A SUPPLEMENT Select a product providing a standardised amount of active constituents, gingerols (eg 15mg).

Ginkgo

WHAT IT IS The Ginkgo Biloba, or Maidenhair tree, has remained virtually unchanged during the last 200 million years. Its fan-shaped leaves contain a variety of unique substances known as ginkgolides and bilobalides.

WHAT IT DOES Ginkgo extracts relax blood vessels and have a thinning action on blood to improve circulation to the brain, hands, feet and genitals. By improving blood flow to the brain, it helps to improve memory, concentration, dizziness, tinnitus, migraine, dementia and some types of depression, while improving blood flow to the rest of the body helps to improve poor peripheral circulation, chilblains, Raynaud's disease, and impotence. It may also be helpful for reducing the risks of deep vein thrombosis on long haul flights.

HOW MUCH YOU NEED Concentrated extracts: 60mg to 120mg daily, either as one dose or divided into three. Concentrated extracts can offer the equivalent of as much as 3000mg fresh ginkgo leaves within just a 60mg tablet.

Effects may not be noticed until after 10 days treatment and may take up to 12 weeks to have a noticeable beneficial effect.

RESEARCH A study involving 40 depressed people aged 51 to 78 years who had not benefited from standard antidepressant drugs found that Ginkgo biloba extracts produced a significant improvement within 8 weeks.

Research shows that Ginkgo biloba can significantly improve memory in older people – the most effective dose seems to be 120mg of extract taken in the morning.

Within one hour of taking Ginkgo biloba, blood flow to the digits is significantly increased by 57% to help overcome cold hands and feet. Over 70% of those taking ginkgo for Raynaud's disease found them helpful.

Ginkgo can improve blood flow to the penis to strengthen and maintain an erection, producing a beneficial effect after 6 - 8 weeks in men with erectile difficulties. After 6 months half of men taking it had regained full potency.

A study involving 50 males with impotence found that all those who had previously relied on injectable drugs to achieve an erection regained potency after taking Ginkgo for 9 months. Of the 30 men who were not helped by medical drugs, 19 regained their erections with ginkgo.

SIDE EFFECTS/SAFETY Seek medical advice before taking Ginkgo if you are taking blood thinning treatment such as warfarin or aspirin, although at usual therapeutic doses of Ginkgo biloba, no effects on blood clotting have been found.

Do not use unprocessed Ginkgo leaves as these contain powerful chemicals that can cause allergic reactions.

Do not take during pregnancy or breast-feeding .

WHAT TO LOOK FOR WHEN SELECTING A SUPPLEMENT Select extracts standardised to provide a known amount of ginkgolides: eg at least 24% flavone glycosides. May be combined with Korean Ginseng for additional benefit.

Hops

WHAT IT IS Hops (Humulus lupulus) are a plant traditionally used to give beer a distinctive, bitter flavour. They contain several unique chemicals such as humulon and lupulin.

WHAT IT DOES Hop flowers are used to stimulate digestion by promoting gastric secretions. They help to quieten over-excitability, and also have antispasmodic and antiseptic actions. Hops are mainly used medicinally for their sedative action that helps to ease tension, anxiety and encourage sleep. They are also used to relieve restlessness, headache and indigestion - conditions which can also cause insomnia.

HOW MUCH YOU NEED 500mg up to 3 times daily.

RESEARCH Hops are thought to reduce activity in some parts of the brain to encourage sleep.

SIDE EFFECTS/SAFETY Do not use if suffering from depression or if you are taking prescribed sleeping tablets. May cause mild drowsiness which will affect your ability to drive or operate machinery.

Do not take during pregnancy or breast-feeding unless advised to by a doctor or medical herbalist.

WHAT TO LOOK FOR WHEN SELECTING A SUPPLEMENT Often combined with lemon balm and valerian for helping insomnia.

Kelp

WHAT IT IS Kelp supplements are obtained from long-leaved seaweeds such as Laminaria and Fucus.

WHAT IT DOES Kelp is a nutritional food source containing 13 vitamins, 20 essential amino acids and 60 minerals and trace elements including calcium, magnesium, potassium, iron and iodine. Its main use is as a source of iodine to improve production of thyroid hormones. It is a popular slimming aid as it contains alginates which promote feelings of fullness. Kelp is also taken to improve quality of hair, skin and nails.

HOW MUCH YOU NEED Depends on product – follow manufacturer's guidelines to obtain the equivalent of 150mcg to 300mcg iodine per day.

RESEARCH Some studies suggest that a kelp-rich diet has a beneficial effect on blood pressure, cholesterol balance and immune function.

SIDE EFFECTS/SAFETY Some people are allergic to iodine, and taking kelp supplements can cause sensitivity reactions. Do not take during pregnancy or breast-feeding unless advised to by a doctor or medical herbalist.

Do not take if you have a thyroid problem without first consulting your doctor.

Korean Ginseng

WHAT IT IS Korean Ginseng (Panax ginseng) is one of the oldest known herbal medicines, used in the Orient as a revitalising tonic for several thousand years. Panax ginseng contains several unique substances, known as ginsenosides, of which 29 have now been identified. Those with a sedative action are mostly derived from small lateral roots, while those with a more stimulating action are mostly derived from the main root.

WHAT IT DOES Ginseng is classed as an adaptogen, which means it helps the body adapt to physical or emotional stress and fatigue. It has a normalising action on many body systems by improving the efficiency with which cells use oxygen, produce energy and clear away waste substances. It is both stimulating and restorative, improving physical and mental energy, stamina, strength, alertness and concentration. It also has a hormone-like action that is beneficial for both men and women. Ginseng is also prized as an aphrodisiac.

Ginseng seems to help support the adrenal glands during times of stress.

HOW MUCH YOU NEED Optimum dose usually around 600mg daily.

Some people prefer to start with a low dose and work up from 200mg to 1200mg per day.

RESEARCH Over 70 international studies have confirmed the beneficial effects of ginseng, including double-blind placebo controlled studies that show benefit in improved energy levels, improved cognition, blood glucose regulation, and immune function.

Ginseng helps the body adapt to physical or emotional stress and fatigue. It is stimulating and restorative, improving physical and mental energy, stamina, strength, alertness and concentration.

A group of hospital nurses who took ginseng were better able to stay awake and perform their night duties than those not taking it.

Men with impotence who took Korean ginseng for 60 days enjoyed significantly improved sexual performance than those taking inactive placebo.

SIDE EFFECTS/SAFETY Should not usually be taken for more than 6 weeks without a break. In the East, ginseng is taken in a two weeks on, two weeks off cycle or in a six weeks on, six weeks off cycle.

Ginseng is not advised if you have high blood pressure (may make hypertension worse), a heart rhythm abnormality, or if you have a hormone dependent condition (eg pregnancy, cancer of the breast, ovaries or uterus).

It is best to avoid taking other stimulants such as caffeine containing products and drinks while taking ginseng.

When taken in therapeutic doses in a two weeks on, two weeks off cycle, side effects should not be a problem. Side effects that have been reported with long-term high doses include sudden high blood pressure, diarrhoea, painful breasts, difficulty sleeping, nervousness, skin eruptions and euphoria. Together, these are known as ginseng abuse syndrome and have occurred in people taking 3g crude root daily for 2 years. Other hormonal effects, such as postmenopausal bleeding and painful breasts (mastalgia) in older women, have also been reported when high doses are taken long term.

Do not take during pregnancy or breast-feeding unless advised to by a doctor or medical herbalist.

WHAT TO LOOK FOR WHEN SELECTING A SUPPLEMENT Select a product supplying a standardised amount of ginsenosides (eg at least 20% or supplying a minimum of 12mg per tablet).

May be combined with Ginkgo biloba for additional benefit.

Lemon balm

WHAT IT IS Lemon balm (Melissa officinalis) is an aromatic herb whose leaves contain a variety of aromatic essential oils.

WHAT IT DOES Lemon balm was known as the "Scholar's Herb" as it was traditionally taken by students suffering from exam stress due to its soothing, calming properties.

It helps relieve a number of stress-related symptoms including digestive problems, nausea, flatulence, depression, tenseness, restlessness, irritability, anxiety, headache and insomnia.

HOW MUCH YOU NEED 650mg up to three times a day

SIDE EFFECTS/SAFETY Do not take if you are using prescribed sleeping tablets. May cause mild drowsiness which will affect your ability to drive or operate machinery.

Do not take during pregnancy or breast-feeding unless advised to by a doctor or medical herbalist.

WHAT TO LOOK FOR WHEN SELECTING A SUPPLEMENT Often combined with valerian and hops for helping insomnia.

Milk thistle

WHAT IT IS Milk thistle (Silybum marianum) is a herb whose seeds contain a unique and powerful mixture of antioxidants known as silymarin, the most active ingredient of which is called silibinin.

WHAT IT DOES Silymarin is mainly used to help protect liver cells from the poisonous effects of excess alcohol. Silymarin is mainly used to treat liver conditions such as hepatitis, cirrhosis, non-obstructive gallstones (by increasing bile flow) and to protect the liver in mushroom poisoning, after chemotherapy, and during detox programs. Silymarin may help the liver metabolise oestrogen more efficiently to reduce symptoms endometriosis. It is also helpful for reducing the excessive skin cell turnover seen in psoriasis.

HOW MUCH YOU NEED 70mg - 200mg silymarin three times a day, preferably between meals.

Concentrated products can contain the equivalent of 3000mg whole herb per 88mg tablet.

RESEARCH Silymarin is a powerful antioxidant and helps to increase levels of an important liver enzyme, glutathione – some studies suggest it increases by as much as one third. It also seems to alter the outer structure of liver cell walls so poisons do not penetrate as easily.

Liver function will start to show an improvement within 5 days and continue over at least the next 3 weeks.

SIDE EFFECTS/SAFETY May cause a mild laxative effect due to increased production of bile.

Do not take during pregnancy or breast-feeding unless advised to by a doctor or medical herbalist.

WHAT TO LOOK FOR WHEN SELECTING A SUPPLEMENT Select products offering a standardised amount of silymarin (eg at least 70% to 80%).

St John's Wort

WHAT IT IS St John's Wort (Hypericum perforatum) is a herb whose petals and leaves contain a number of unique substances such as hypericin, pseudohypericin and hyperforin.

WHAT IT DOES St John's Wort is used as a natural antidepressant that is thought to work by prolonging the action of a brain neurotransmitter, serotonin. St John's Wort increases nocturnal production of melatonin hormone (the brains natural sedative), to improve the quality of sleep. Hypericum is also helpful for seasonal affective disorder.

HOW MUCH YOU NEED 300mg three times a day. One a day formulations also available.

RESEARCH Studies involving over 5000 people shows that Hypericum can lift mild depression within two weeks of starting the course - and the optimum effect is reached within six weeks. Three out of four people showed a marked improvement after only five weeks, with one in three becoming symptom-free.

Studies involving 263 people found that St John's Wort extracts providing 900mcg hypericin daily were at least as effective as taking 100mg imipramine (a tricyclic anti-depressant) in treating moderate depression but with less risk of side effects.

When compared with sertraline, a prescribed antidepressant drug, standardised extracts of St John's Wort were at least as effective in the treatment of mild to moderate depression.

Research involving 111 post-menopausal women (aged 45-65 years) with low sex drive plus physical exhaustion found that taking Hypericum for three months helped 60% regain their sex drive. Eighty-two per cent also suffered less irritability, anxiety, low mood, hot flushes, sweating and disturbed sleep.

SIDE EFFECTS/SAFETY St John's Wort is best taken with food. Avoid alcohol.

Side effects of indigestion, allergic reactions, restlessness and tiredness each affect less than 1% of people.

Avoid direct skin exposure to sunlight especially if fair-skinned.

Do not take together with other antidepressant drugs. Other interactions currently recognised between Hypericum perforatum and prescribed drugs are with warfarin, cyclosporin, oral contraceptives, anticonvulsants, digoxin, theophylline, HIV protease inhibitors, triptans and SSRI anti-depressants.

Do not take during pregnancy or breast-feeding unless advised to by a doctor or medical herbalist.

WHAT TO LOOK FOR WHEN SELECTING A SUPPLEMENT Select extracts supplying a standardised amount of hypericin (eg 0.3% or 900mcg); one-a-day formulas are also available.

Saw palmetto

WHAT IT IS The saw palmetto (Sabal serrulata, Serenoa repens) is a small palm tree whose fruit contains hormone-like substances known as sterols.

WHAT IT DOES Saw Palmetto is mainly used to help symptoms due to an enlarged male prostate gland (benign prostatic hyperplasia or BPH) which causes urinary hesitancy, frequency, urgency and poor flow. Saw palmetto fruit extracts seem to help the central part of the prostate gland shrink, so the urinary tube which passes through is less constricted. It also helps the prostate gland relax, to reduce spasm, and also seems to normalise hormone actions within the gland.

Saw palmetto is also used in women with polycystic ovary syndrome, but should only be taken by females under the supervision of a medical herbalist.

HOW MUCH YOU NEED 160-320mg daily – may be divided into two separate doses. A beneficial effect usually starts within two to six weeks.

RESEARCH A study of 176 patients showed significant improvement in both day and night time urinary frequency plus a significant increase in urinary flow rate after taking saw palmetto extracts for 60 days.

A meta-analysis which assessed results from 18 studies involving 2939 men found that Saw palmetto fruit extracts improved urinary tract symptoms by 28%, night time frequency by 25%, urinary flow by 28% and reduced the amount of urine remaining in the bladder after voiding by 43%.

In trials where saw palmetto extracts were compared with a variety of drugs prescribed to improve prostate symptoms, the herbal extracts were found to be at least as effective - but with fewer unwanted side effects such as erectile dysfunction. A trial comparing extracts of saw palmetto with a prescription-only drug (finasteride), for example, showed both treatments achieved a 38% decrease in symptoms over a 6 month period. Sexual function in the men using Saw palmetto did not change, although it deteriorated significantly in those taking the prescribed drug.

SIDE EFFECTS/SAFETY No significant side effects reported. Do not take during pregnancy or breast-feeding.

WHAT TO LOOK FOR WHEN SELECTING A SUPPLEMENT Select products supplying a standardised amount of free fatty acids/fat soluble sterols (eg 80%).

May be combined with zinc and evening primrose oil for additional benefit.

Valerian

WHAT IT IS Valerian (Valerian officinalis) is a calming herb whose roots contain a number of unique substances such as valeric acid, valepotriates, that have a sedative action.

WHAT IT DOES Valerian is used to help calm nervous anxiety, stress, muscle tension, to stimulate appetite and promote a refreshing night's sleep. It is also used to relieve cramps, period pains, intestinal colic, irritable bowel syndrome, migraine and rheumatic pains.

HOW MUCH YOU NEED 250mg – 800mg two to three times a day. For sleeping, take thirty minutes before going to bed. Concentrated extracts can provide the equivalent of 250mg valerian root per 50mg extract (5:1).

RESEARCH Valerian has been shown to help reduce low mood, loss of initiative, feeling unsociable, irritability, anxiety and difficulty sleeping in people under stress.

A study involving 125 people found those taking valerian extracts fell asleep more quickly and woke up less often during the night than those taking placebo.

A study involving 16 patients with insomnia found that 300mg concentrated dry extract (equivalent to 1800mg fresh herb) produced beneficial effects on slow wave sleep latency and duration.

Valerian is thought to work by raising levels of an inhibitory brain chemical (GABA) which damps down the over-stimulation occurring during anxiety.

SIDE EFFECTS/SAFETY May cause mild drowsiness which will affect your ability to drive or operate machinery. Valerian is not addictive, and does not produce a drugged feeling or hangover effect, as it promotes a natural form of sleep whose architecture is preserved.

Do not take if you are using prescribed sleeping tablets. Do not take during pregnancy or breast-feeding.

WHAT TO LOOK FOR WHEN SELECTING A SUPPLEMENT Select products containing a standardised amount of valeric or valerenic acid (eg 0.8%).

Often combined with lemon balm and hops for helping insomnia.

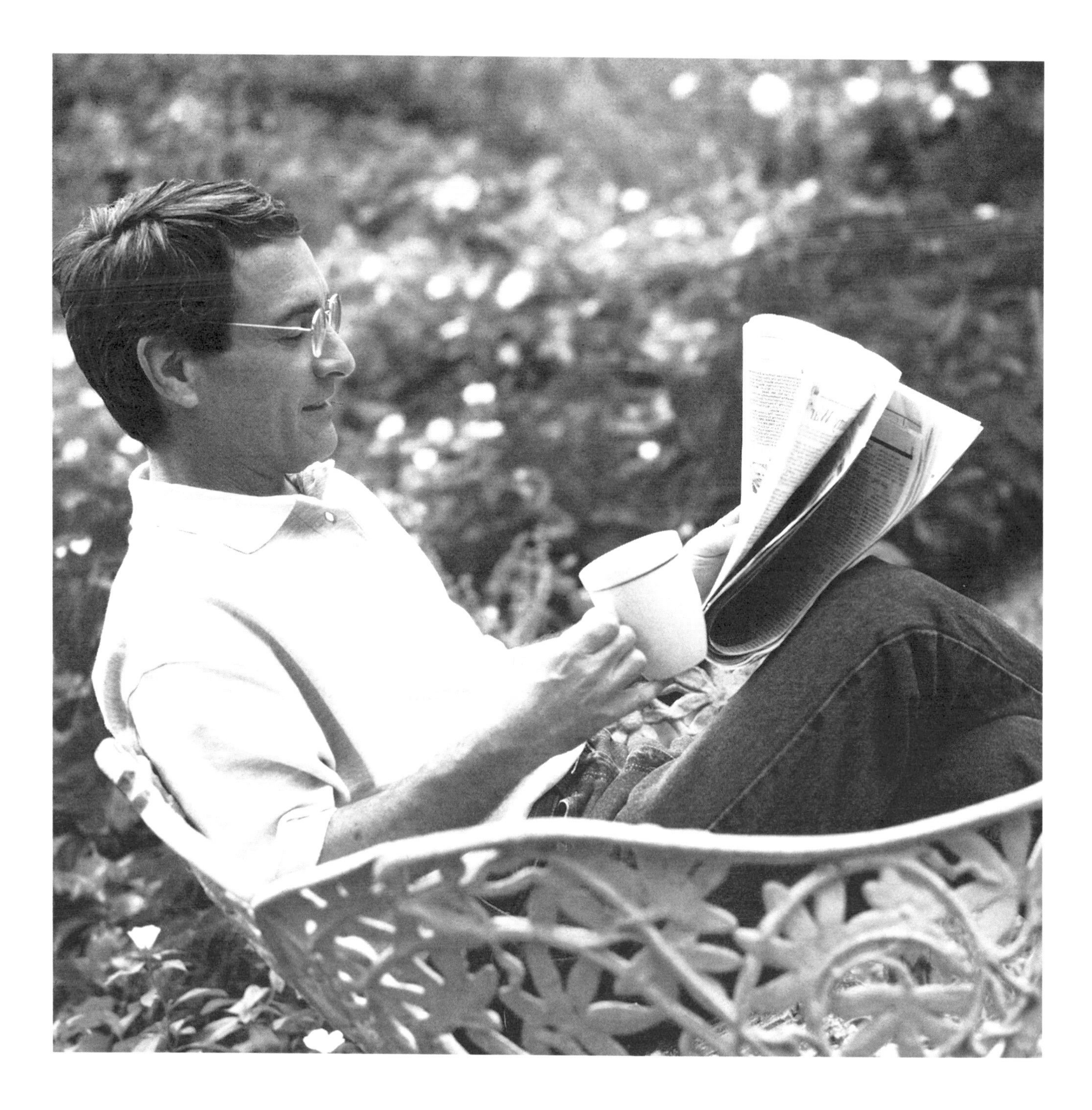

Section Six: The other important Food supplements

Alpha lipoic acid

WHAT IT IS Alpha-lipoic acid (ALA) is a vitamin like substance. The body produces small quantities of alpha-lipoic acid, and some is also obtained from the diet (eg in spinach, meats).

WHAT IT DOES ALA acts as a co-enzyme with B group vitamins to speed metabolic reactions involved in energy production in cells. It is a powerful antioxidant and regenerates other important antioxidants such as vitamins C and E. Alpha-lipoic acid is mainly used to boost energy levels, and reduce chronic fatigue. It is also taken to help treat symptoms linked with nerve damage such as tingling, numbness or discomfort, and liver problems such as hepatitis and cirrhosis

HOW MUCH YOU NEED 50 to 100mg daily as an antioxidant. 100 to 200mg up to three times a day for therapeutic use.

RESEARCH Recent research suggests that taking 200mg ALA plus 250mg L-carnitine caused animals to appear to become significantly younger in a number of different measures of ageing, including memory and energy levels.

SIDE EFFECTS/SAFETY Mild skin rashes or gastrointestinal side effects have occurred, but are rare.

WHAT TO LOOK FOR WHEN SELECTING A SUPPLEMENT Alpha-lipoic acid, L-Carnitine and coenzyme Q10 seem to work synergistically and are often taken together.

Betacarotene

WHAT IT IS Betacarotene is a yellow, carotenoid pigment found in dark green, leafy vegetables and yellow-orange fruits. It is made up of two molecules of vitamin A joined together and can be split to yield vitamin A. Nutritionally, 6mcg betacarotene is equivalent to around 1mcg of preformed retinol.

- ✖ Canning vegetables loses 20% - 35% betacarotene content
- ✖ Drying fruit and vegetables loses up to 20% - open air drying loses all vitamin A activity

WHAT IT DOES Betacarotene acts as an antioxidant, and as a source of vitamin A. On average, we convert around half of the betacarotene we eat into vitamin A. Betacarotene forms an important part of our carotenoid intake, working together with other antioxidants to produce beneficial effects against coronary heart disease and possibly some cancers.

HOW MUCH YOU NEED 6mg to 15mg daily as part of a mixed carotenoid intake.

RESEARCH Several studies suggest that natural dietary intakes of betacarotene and vitamin A are important in reducing the risk of coronary heart disease and a number of cancers. Whether supplemental forms can do the same remains unclear. Some of the research benefits of a betacarotene-rich diet may be due to other carotenoids present in fruit and vegetables which are now known to have important antioxidant activity in their own right..

SIDE EFFECTS/SAFETY Supplemental forms of betacarotene are best avoided by those who smoke. One trial found that people with a high risk of lung cancer through smoking did not benefit from taking betacarotene supplements, and the risks may even have been increased.

Excess causes a yellow-orange discolouration of skin, which resolves when intakes are reduced.

WHAT TO LOOK FOR WHEN SELECTING A SUPPLEMENT Best taken in balance with other mixed carotenoids (eg alphacarotene, cryptoxanthin, zeaxanthin, lutein) for maximum benefit.

May be combined with other antioxidants, including vitamins C and E, for optimum antioxidant protection.

Co-enzyme Q10

WHAT IT IS Co-enzyme Q10 (CoQ10) is a vitamin-like substance also known as ubiquinone.

Levels of CoQ10 start to decrease over the age of 20 years as we absorb less CoQ10 from our diet and produce less in body cells. As a result, cells do not receive all the energy they need, which has been linked with premature ageing. Dietary sources include meat, fish, wholegrains, nuts and green vegetables.

WHAT IT DOES CoQ10 improves oxygen uptake and use during energy production in cells.

CoQ10 acts together with vitamin E to protect body fats from oxidation, and helps to reduce the risk of hardening and furring up of the arteries (atherosclerosis) and coronary heart disease. It is also helpful for those with Raynaud's disease, and may play a role in weight loss. CoQ10 also helps to protect against gum disease.

Recent research suggests that co-enzyme Q10 can slow disease progression in people with early stage Parkinson's disease. While the results must be confirmed in a larger study, they provide hope that CoQ10 may ultimately provide a new way of treating Parkinson's disease.

HOW MUCH YOU NEED Supplements range from 10mg to 100mg daily. Higher amounts of 600mg may be taken for therapeutic use.

CoQ10 is best taken with food to improve absorption as it is fat soluble. It usually takes at least three weeks and occasionally up to three months before the full beneficial effect and extra energy levels are noticed.

RESEARCH Research suggests falling CoQ10 levels play a significant role in age-related medical conditions such as coronary heart disease. Biopsies of heart muscle from patients with various forms of heart disease have shown that over half are deficient in CoQ10.

CoQ10 is used by some doctors to treat patients with coronary heart disease and in heart failure.

People taking a type of drug called a statin, designed to lower cholesterol levels, should consider taking CoQ10 supplements, as statins reduce levels of CoQ10.

A study of 18 people with high blood pressure found that taking 100mg CoQ10 daily significantly reduce blood pressure by an average of 10.6/7.7 mmHg when taking CoQ10, but did not change with placebo. CoQ10 is thought to lower hypertension by improving the elasticity and reactivity of the blood vessel wall.

CoQ10 may be useful in weight loss by stimulating fat burning in cells. When two groups of people with obesity followed a controlled reducing diet, those taking CoQ10 for nine weeks lost an average of 30 pounds, compared with an average of 13 pounds for the other group.

SIDE EFFECTS/SAFETY No serious side effects have been reported, even at high dose - only occasional, mild nausea.

WHAT TO LOOK FOR WHEN SELECTING A SUPPLEMENT CoQ10 is better absorbed in an oil based capsule rather than in tablet form. Tablet forms may be preferable to vegetarians, however.

To use CoQ10 to the full, you also need to ensure a good intake of B and C vitamins.

Chondroitin

WHAT IT IS Chondroitin sulphate is made up of a chain of sugars (galactosamine sulphate and glucuronic acid) to which sulphate groups are attached. It is closely related to glucosamine (see page 76) and is usually combined with it for additional benefit.

WHAT IT DOES Chondroitin sulphate supplies building blocks for making structural substances known as glycosaminoglycans (GAGs) in joints. It attracts water into joints, which acts as a shock absorber as well as a nutrient transport system. Chondroitin sulphate inhibits enzymes that break down cartilage, while stimulating those involved in the production of structural substances such as proteoglycans, glycosaminoglycans and collagen. Chondroitin sulphate helps to raise blood levels of hyaluronan, a sticky gel that cements joint tissues together.

Clinical studies show that taking chondroitin sulphate plus glucosamine sulphate have a beneficial action to reduce pain, swelling and restore mobility in people with arthritic joints. It has also been shown to inhibit hardening and furring up of the arteries.

HOW MUCH YOU NEED Optimum intake may be 800mg to 1600mg depending on body weight.

Most people with joint problems would probably benefit from 1,500mg. glucosamine plus 1,200mg. chondroitin sulphate, although lower intakes of 250-500mg chondroitin sulphate per day have also produced benefits in trials.

It may be helpful to divide the dose into 2 to 4 doses taken during the day.

RESEARCH A study of 50 people with osteoarthritis of the knee showed that after taking chondroitin sulphate for three months, their cartilage showed more evidence of repair than in those taking placebo.

A study found that people with osteoarthritis who took chondroitin sulphate were able to reduce their use of pain-killing anti-inflammatory drugs by almost halve.

146 people with osteoarthritis of the knee were given either chondroitin sulphate or the pain-killing anti-inflammatory drug, diclofenac. Those treated with diclofenac showed prompt reduction of clinical symptoms but these reappeared after the end of treatment. Those taking chondroitin sulphate took longer to achieve pain reduction, but results lasted for up to 3 months after the end of treatment.

Other studies have shown a significant decrease in the number of people with new erosive findings in finger joints on x-ray, and a significant reduction in joint space narrowing in those taking chondroitin sulphate compared with those on placebo.

SIDE EFFECTS/SAFETY No significant side effects reported.

WHAT TO LOOK FOR WHEN SELECTING A SUPPLEMENT Consider whether or not you would prefer to select products providing marine chondroitin sourced exclusively from fish, rather than bovine chondroitin sourced from cattle.

Best taken together with glucosamine sulphate and a multinutrient that includes vitamin C, manganese and copper.

Glucosamine

WHAT IT IS Glucosamine sulphate is a substance that is naturally made in the body from a sugar (glucose) and an amino acid (glutamine). Larger quantities are needed when damaged joints are healing and, as production of glucosamine is normally a slow process, it is often in short supply.

WHAT IT DOES Glucosamine sulphate is needed in the body to produce molecules (glycosaminoglycans) for laying down new framework tissues in damaged joints. It is essential for the production of new cartilage and synthesis of the joint's oil (synovial fluid), helping to make it thicker and more cushioning. It strengthens the jelly-like centre of intervertebral discs and is also needed for healthy formation of nails, tendons, skin, eyes, bone, ligaments and mucous membranes.

HOW MUCH YOU NEED 1000mg - 2000mg daily (depending on body weight) in divided doses.

RESEARCH Glucosamine sulphate can improve joint symptoms associated with sports injuries and arthritis by at least 40% and often up to 70% compared with an inactive placebo.

A landmark clinical trial compared the effects of glucosamine sulphate (1500mg once daily for three years) versus placebo, on the long-term progression of knee osteoarthritis in 212 patients. Those taking placebo showed progressive narrowing of the knee joint space over the 3 year trial period, while those taking glucosamine sulphate showed no significant loss of joint space. Those receiving glucosamine sulphate enjoyed significant improvements in pain and disability which was sustained for the 3 year duration of the trial; in contrast, those taking the placebo experienced a significant worsening of symptoms. The authors concluded that 'The long-term structure-modifying and symptom-modifying effects of glucosamine sulphate suggest that it could be a disease modifying agent in osteoarthritis'.

Glucosamine sulphate appears to be at least as effective in reducing joint pain as non-steroidal anti-inflammatory painkillers such as ibuprofen. In a study involving 178 people with osteoarthritis of the knee, those taking glucosamine 1500mg daily for 4 weeks showed improvements similar to those seen with ibuprofen 1200mg daily, but with less side effects. Two weeks after stopping treatment, those who had taken glucosamine had a better residual therapeutic effect than those taking the non-steroidal anti-inflammatory drug.

SIDE EFFECTS/SAFETY No significant side effects reported. It should not be used in pregnancy as it's effects have not yet been investigated.

WHAT TO LOOK FOR WHEN SELECTING A SUPPLEMENT Glucosamine sulphate seems to be the optimum form of glucosamine, as opposed to N-acetyl-glucosamine as it has the best research data to support its use.

Most people would benefit from 1,500mg. glucosamine plus 1,200mg. chondroitin sulphate.

Best taken together with a multinutrient that includes vitamin C, manganese and copper which help to stimulate collagen production.

Green Lipped Mussels

WHAT IT IS Green-lipped mussels (Perna canaliculus) grow in the unique marine conditions found around parts of New Zealand.

WHAT IT DOES Raw extracts contain substances that help to reduce inflammation in joints. It is mainly used to help reduce symptoms of rheumatoid arthritis and osteo arthritis.

HOW MUCH YOU NEED 1,000-1,250mg

RESEARCH Some studies have failed to show a benefit, while others suggest it has an effective anti-inflammatory action equivalent to that of non-steroidal anti-inflammatory pain killers (eg ibuprofen), possibly by helping to prevent inflammatory white blood cells moving into the joints.

In a trial involving 86 patients, around two thirds of those with rheumatoid arthritis and one third of those with osteoarthritis experienced reduced pain, stiffness and joint inflammation.

SIDE EFFECTS/SAFETY May cause nausea, flatulence, gout and skin rashes.

Do not take if you have a shell fish allergy.

WHAT TO LOOK FOR WHEN SELECTING A SUPPLEMENT Extracts stabilised with a preservative may be more effective.

L-Carnitine

WHAT IT IS L-carnitine is a non-essential amino acid that is made in the liver. It is also found in the diet especially in red meats, offal and dairy products. Vegetable sources of L-carnitine are avocado and the fermented soybean product, tempeh.

WHAT IT DOES L-carnitine is needed to regulate fat metabolism by transporting long chain fatty acids to the energy producing apparatus (mitochondria) in cells. The more L-carnitine there is available, the more fat can be burned, especially in exercising muscle such as heart muscle. L-carnitine is also needed to break down the branched-chain amino acids (leucine, isoleucine and valine) so they can be used as an emergency energy source. By mobilising fat stores and boosting energy production, L-carnitine may play a useful role in weight loss, improving the appearance of cellulite, and lowering cholesterol and triglyceride levels. It also stimulates secretion of gastric and pancreatic juices to aid digestion.

HOW MUCH YOU NEED 250mg to 1g daily.

RESEARCH Recent research suggests that taking 200mg ALA plus 250mg L-carnitine caused animals to appear to become significantly younger in a number of different measures of ageing, including memory and energy levels.

Taking L- carnitine may help to minimise heart damage in those at risk of a heart attack. A study of 44 men with angina found almost a quarter of those taking L-carnitine supplements for four weeks became free of exercise-induced angina compared with only 9% taking placebo.

L-Carnitine improves the distance walked without pain in patients with calf pain due to poor peripheral circulation. One study found it increased pain-free walking distance by 75% after three weeks.

In 18 people with chronic fatigue, L-carnitine helped two thirds experience less tiredness and muscle weakness within 4 to 8 weeks.

100 men with low fertility who took L-carnitine experienced a significant improvement in sperm quality and quantity.

SIDE EFFECTS/SAFETY Increased body odour and diarrhoea may occur at very high doses (eg over 4g daily).

WHAT TO LOOK FOR WHEN SELECTING A SUPPLEMENT Alpha-lipoic acid, L-Carnitine and coenzyme Q10 seem to work synergistically and are often taken together.

Lecithin

WHAT IT IS Lecithin is a type of fat known as a phospholipid, and its chemical name is phosphatidyl choline. It is a rich source of choline and inositol. Lecithin is now known to be an essential dietary component which cannot be made in the body in quantities high enough to meet our needs.

Thirty years ago, the average Western diet supplied around 6,000mg lecithin daily. Modern low fat eating has reduced this significantly, however. One egg supplies around 2000mg lecithin.

WHAT IT DOES Lecithin provides building blocks to make healthy cell membranes, and for healthy nerve and brain function. It helps to reduce the risk of coronary heart disease by lowering cholesterol levels as a result of inhibiting intestinal absorption of cholesterol, and by increasing the excretion of cholesterol and bile acids. Lecithin is also important for liver function and helps to prevent a build up of fats in liver cells. It is an essential component of bile and keeps cholesterol emulsified to reduce gallstone formation. The choline found within lecithin is converted into acetylcholine, an important brain chemical needed for passing messages between brain cells.

HOW MUCH YOU NEED 1g to 10g daily. A good daily intake is 1200mg to 4800mg daily.

One tablespoon of lecithin granules provides 1,725mg phosphatidylcholine and 250mg choline, a little less than provided by a hen's egg. Best taken with meals to boost absorption.

RESEARCH A study of 32 people with high blood fat levels showed that taking 10.5g lecithin for 30 days reduced average total cholesterol and triglycerides decreased by one-third. Harmful LDL cholesterol decreased by 38% while beneficial HDL cholesterol increased by 46%.

Lecithin is also needed for healthy nerve-cell growth and function, and appears to have beneficial effects on memory.

Lecithin helps to reverse fatty build up in liver cells of people with fatty liver disease and may help to protect against liver change in people with excessive alcohol intakes.

61 healthy people aged 50 to 80 years took either lecithin or placebo for five weeks. Memory tests in those taking lecithin were significantly improved compared with those taking placebo. Those taking lecithin also reported a 48% reduction in memory lapses.

Lecithin and choline supplements have been shown to improve athletic performance – perhaps by improving communication between nerve and muscle fibres.

SIDE EFFECTS/SAFETY Supplements should not be taken by those with manic depression except under medical supervision in case it makes their condition worse.

WHAT TO LOOK FOR WHEN SELECTING A SUPPLEMENT Ideally take with vitamin B5 to improve their effect in the body.

Lycopene

WHAT IT IS Lycopene is a carotenoid that is best known as the red pigment in tomatoes. Cooking tomatoes releases five times more lycopene than is available from raw tomatoes. Lycopene makes up at least 50% of all carotenoids found in the human body.

WHAT IT DOES Lycopene is a powerful antioxidant. Increasing research suggests that, of the many types of carotenoids found in food, lycopene is the most beneficial for protecting against coronary heart disease and cancer. Lycopene is also important for eye health.

HOW MUCH YOU NEED 250mg standardised tomato extract provides 15mg lycopene – equivalent to at least six, large, ripe tomatoes.

RESEARCH Lycopene may play an important protective role in cardiovascular disease. In one study, 19 young men followed a diet based on tomato juice, spaghetti sauce and other tomato-based products. Their cholesterol levels were then measured and compared to that of 20 men following their normal diet. In those eating more tomatoes, there was a significant increase in blood lycopene levels which in turn reduced the amount of harmful LDL-cholesterol that became oxidised (chemical change to the cholesterol that is thought to increase the risk of coronary heart disease).

An analysis of 72 studies found that 57 studies reported significant links between tomato intake or blood lycopene levels and reduced risk of cancer, especially of the lung, stomach, mouth, colon, rectum and prostate gland.

After accounting for smoking, people with the lowest levels of lycopene are three times more likely to develop lung cancer than those with the highest intakes.

In one six-year study, men who ate two or more servings of tomato products a week, reduced their risk of prostate cancer by up to 50%. A family history of prostate cancer did not seem to reduce the protective effect of lycopene. Another study found that men with the highest lycopene levels were up to 60% less likely to develop prostate cancer than those with the lowest blood levels.

Laboratory experiments suggest that when lycopene and vitamin E act together, prostate cancer cells are stopped from growing and multiplying by as much as 90%.

Women with the highest lycopene levels appear to have five times less chance of developing an abnormal cervical smear than women with low lycopene levels.

Lycopene was recently shown to be depleted in skin exposed to ultraviolet light, suggesting that it plays a role in protecting the skin from sun damage.

People with the lowest levels of lycopene have been shown to have more than double the risk of developing macular degeneration of the eyes – one of the leading causes of reduced vision in older people.

SIDE EFFECTS/SAFETY No significant side effects reported.

WHAT TO LOOK FOR WHEN SELECTING A SUPPLEMENT Combine with other antioxidants such as vitamins C, E and selenium for optimum benefit.

Lutein

WHAT IT IS Lutein is a carotenoid pigment which acts as an antioxidant. It cannot be made in the body and must therefore come from the diet. Good sources of lutein include yellow-orange and dark green fruit and vegetables, such as sweetcorn, pumpkin, spinach and broccoli. It is also found in egg yolk.

WHAT IT DOES Lutein is important for healthy vision. The macula of the eye contains two carotenoids, lutein and zeaxanthin, which can be made from lutein. Lutein helps to protect the macular degeneration which affects as many as 20 percent of people aged over 65 and is the leading cause of visual loss. As an antioxidant, lutein neutralises harmful free radicals generated during the chemical processes of light detection, while its yellow colour filters out visible blue light, which can cause photodamage to the retina. It is often referred to as nature's sunglasses. High intakes of lutein and zeaxanthin may decrease the risk of cataracts, coronary heart disease and lung cancer.

HOW MUCH YOU NEED 6mg to 20mg daily

RESEARCH Those who consume the most lutein-containing foods are likely to have thick macular pigments and a low risk of macular degeneration. People with macular degeneration have, on average, 70% less lutein and zeaxanthin in their eyes than those with health vision.

In one study, in which two people took 30mg lutein supplements per day, their macular density increased by 21% and 39% after 20 weeks. Even after lutein was discontinued, their maculae continued to improve for about six weeks.

A study involving 8 people with early macular degeneration and 8 with normal vision found that taking lutein supplements for 12 weeks caused a similar rate of increase in macular pigment in both groups. Also, where a person had macular degeneration in only one eye, both eyes responded equally well to supplementation.

This suggests that already having early age-related macular degeneration does not stop lutein from being deposited in the retina which might help to prevent the condition progressing.

A study involving almost 77,500 female nurses aged 45-71 years found that, after age, smoking, and other potential cataract risk factors were controlled for, those with the highest intake of lutein and zeaxanthin were 22% less likely to develop cataracts severe enough to require extraction.

SIDE EFFECTS/SAFETY No significant side effects reported. High doses may cause temporary (and harmless) orange-discoloration of the skin. High doses of carotenoids should be avoided during pregnancy.

MSM-Sulphur

WHAT IT IS MSM (methyl-sulphonyl-methane) is a sulphur compound that is made naturally in the body from the amino acids, methionine, cysteine and taurine.

WHAT IT DOES Like glucosamine sulphate (see page 78) MSM is important for healthy joints, cartilage, tendons and ligaments. MSM is used to help a number of conditions, including allergies, acid indigestion, constipation, and degenerative bone diseases. It is vital for production of healthy connective tissue as it is a major building block needed to make glycosaminoglycans – the key structural component of collagen. MSM may also help to maintain suppleness of tissues in later life.

HOW MUCH YOU NEED 1g to 2.5g daily, in divided doses. It seems to be beneficial to start with 1600mg daily, for a week, increasing to 2400mg daily thereafter. After two months, you can reduce back down to 1600mg daily.

RESEARCH A trial involving 16 people with osteoarthritis found that those taking MSM experienced an 82% reduction in joint pain after six weeks, compared with an average improvement of only 18% in those on placebo.

SIDE EFFECTS/SAFETY Excess may produce gastrointestinal side effects. Best taken with meals.

WHAT TO LOOK FOR WHEN SELECTING A SUPPLEMENT MSM and glucosamine seem to work together and you may therefore want to take them both.

Probiotics

WHAT IT IS **Pro**biotics is the use of natural 'friendly' lactic acid producing bacteria such as Lactobacilli and Bifidobacteria naturally found in the large bowel to encourage a healthy digestive balance.

A similar word, **Pre**biotics describes the use of food substances such as fructo-oligosaccharides (FOS) and oatmeal that promote the growth of probiotic bacteria, and which encourage colonisation of the bowel with friendly microbes. FOS cannot be digested or absorbed from the human bowel, but act as a fermentable food source for probiotic bacteria in the gut. In contrast, harmful bacteria such as E. coli and Clostridium cannot use FOS as a source of energy. Dietary sources of FOS include garlic, onions, barley, wheat, bananas, honey and tomatoes.

Synbiotics is the term used when both prebiotic and probiotic supplements are taken together.

WHAT IT DOES Probiotic bacteria produce lactic acid, which helps to create a healthy intestinal environment and discourage infection with potentially harmful, disease-causing organisms (viral, bacterial and fungal) known as pathogens. Probiotic bacteria improve intestinal health, promote good digestion, boost immunity and increase resistance to infection - especially during foreign travel. They are especially helpful for people with intestinal problems such as irritable bowel syndrome and inflammatory bowel disease (Crohn's and ulcerative colitis).

Lactobacilli are also needed for optimum vaginal health and to protect against recurrent Candida infections, and bacterial vaginosis (a condition in which healthy vaginal Lactobacilli are severely depleted).

HOW MUCH YOU NEED 1 to 5 billion colony forming units daily.

RESEARCH Probiotic bacteria have been shown to reduce overgrowth of harmful pathogens in the intestines in a number of different ways, including:

- the production of lactic and acetic acids which discourages growth of potentially harmful bacteria including those responsible for traveller's diarrhoea
- secreting natural antibiotics known as bacteriocins, and stimulating production of interferon, a natural substance that helps to protect against viral infections
- competing with harmful bacteria and yeasts for available nutrients
- competing with other bacteria for attachment site on intestinal cell walls - literally crowding them out so they pass through the intestines without gaining a foothold.

These actions have been shown to help reduce the risk and severity of bacterial food poisoning caused by Bacillus cereus, Salmonella typhi, Shigella dysenteriae, Escherichia coli and Staphylococcus aureus, as well as reducing the side effects (eg diarrhoea) caused by taking antibiotics

A study of 100 people with irritable bowel syndrome found that taking probiotic bacteria produced a 75% improvement in symptoms compared with 30% in those taking the anti-spasm drug, mebeverine. When Lactobacilli were taking with mebeverine, improvements increased to 90%. No improvement occurred in those taking an inactivated placebo solution of lactobacilli.

Research suggests bowel bacteria have a modulating effect on the immune system, helping to reduce the risk of allergies such as eczema.

SIDE EFFECTS/SAFETY No significant side effects reported.

WHAT TO LOOK FOR WHEN SELECTING A SUPPLEMENT Select a supplement supplying a known quantity of probiotic bacteria (eg 5 billion colony forming units (CFU) per dose).

Check whether or not your supplement needs refrigeration. Most do. A few made using a modern micro-encapsulation process helps to protect both shelf life and the ability of the bacteria to pass through the stomach into the lower intestines.

Psyllium

WHAT IT IS Psyllium seed and husks from the plant species, Plantago (eg Plantago ovata, also known as blonde psyllium), are a highly effective, natural and gentle fibre source.

WHAT IT DOES Psyllium is widely used to help treat bowel problems such as constipation and irritable bowel syndrome. Many people do not eat the recommended 18g to 30g fibre per day, and a fibre supplement is often a good idea to help maintain bowel regularity. In the intestines, psyllium forms a laxative bulk that acts rather like a sponge, gently scrubbing the bowel clean as well as absorbing toxins and excess fats. Psyllium can absorb between 10 and 20 times its own weight in water and waste material in the bowels. It is particularly helpful for people who cannot tolerate other forms of fibre such as bran.

Fibre also binds cholesterol and other fats in the bowel to reduce their absorption and can have a significant effect on cholesterol levels.

HOW MUCH YOU NEED 10g daily.

RESEARCH Psyllium contains mucilage, which swells to between 8 and 14 times its original volume when mixed with water.

Taking just 10g psyllium seed daily for at least six weeks can reduce LDL-cholesterol levels by between 5% and 20%.

A group of people with ulcerative colitis who were given psyllium husk fibre supplements during remission were found to have significantly greater improvement than those not taking them.

SIDE EFFECTS/SAFETY Drink plenty of water when taking fibre supplements to help them swell up and work properly.

Fibre supplements – especially psyllium – should not be taken within two hours of any prescribed medication as it may interfere with its absorption.

Pycnogenol

WHAT IT IS Pycnogenol is an extract obtained from the bark of the French maritime pine. It contains a rich blend of natural fruit acids and antioxidants.

WHAT IT DOES Pine bark extracts have a beneficial effect on the circulation, reducing hardening and furring up of the arteries, thinning the blood, reducing clumping of clotting fragments (platelets) and reducing the risk of coronary heart disease and stroke. It is widely taken to treat conditions associated with poor circulation, such as diabetes, impotence, varicose veins, thread veins, macular degeneration, peripheral vascular disease, intermittent claudication and leg cramps. It is also used to reduce the risk of DVT on long haul flights by those unable to take aspirin as it does not produce side effects of stomach irritation, peptic ulcers or gastric bleeding as can occur with aspirin therapy.

HOW MUCH YOU NEED 30mg to 200mg daily. May be divided into two doses.

RESEARCH Research suggests that, as an antioxidant, pycnogenol is 50 times more powerful than vitamin E, 20 times more powerful than vitamin C and 16 times more active than grapeseed extracts.

Preliminary studies suggest pycnogenol is as effective at reducing abnormal blood clotting in smokers as aspirin. 125mg pycnogenol is as effective in preventing increased susceptibility to clotting as 500mg aspirin, but without the increased stomach-bleeding time seem with aspirin.

SIDE EFFECTS/SAFETY No significant side effects reported.

WHAT TO LOOK FOR WHEN SELECTING A SUPPLEMENT As pine bark extracts enhance the effects of other antioxidants such as Co-enzyme Q10, vitamin C and E, they are often combined in supplements.

Royal jelly

WHAT IT IS Royal jelly is a milky-white substance secreted by the salivary glands of worker honey bees. It is a highly concentrated food given to all larvae for the first three days of their lives. After that, only the larva destined to become a queen bee will continue to receive Royal jelly.

WHAT IT DOES Royal jelly is one of the richest natural sources of vitamin B5 (pantothenic acid), and also contains other B vitamins plus vitamins A, C, D, and E, 20 amino acids, essential fatty acids, minerals such as potassium, calcium, zinc, iron and manganese. It is such a nutritious energy source, the queen bee grows 50% larger than other genetically-identical female bees and has a lifespan nearly 40 times longer. Royal jelly is traditionally taken to boost energy levels, mental alertness and to combat stress, fatigue, and insomnia. As a tonic, it is said to boost feelings of well-being, increase vitality – especially after illness - improve the complexion and help to maintain healthy skin, hair and nails. Royal Jelly also contains acetylcholine, essential for passing messages from one nerve cell to another, plus inositol which helps emulsify fats and may reduce cholesterol levels.

HOW MUCH YOU NEED 50 to 600mg daily. Concentrated supplements can contain the equivalent of 600mg fresh Royal Jelly per 200mg capsule (3:1). Best taken on an empty stomach.

RESEARCH Royal jelly contains an antibiotic, referred to as royalisin, which is effective against certain skin bacteria.

Royal jelly may help to protect against hardening and furring up of the arteries (atherosclerosis) by lowering total blood fats and abnormal cholesterol levels.

Royal jelly has been shown to decrease blood cholesterol levels by 14 percent and total serum lipids by 10 percent.

SIDE EFFECTS/SAFETY Royal jelly has been known to trigger severe asthma attacks in some people with asthma so do not take if you are allergic to bee products, or if you suffer from asthma or other allergic conditions.

WHAT TO LOOK FOR WHEN SELECTING A SUPPLEMENT Usually blended with honey or freeze-dried to preserve its active ingredients.

Soy Isoflavones

WHAT IT IS Isoflavones (eg genistein, daidzein, formononetin, biochanin A, glycitein) found in members of the pea and bean family such as soya and chickpeas.

WHAT IT DOES Isoflavones are plant substances with a weak, oestrogen-like action in the body.

They help to damp down high oestrogen states by competing for the stronger natural oestrogens at oestrogen receptors. This reduces the amount of oestrogen stimulation a cell receives. As they have a weak oestrogen action, phytoestrogens also provide a useful additional hormone boost when oestrogen levels are low after the menopause.

They therefore act as a natural form of hormone replacement therapy.

Isoflavones help to dilate coronary arteries, increase heart function, reduce blood levels of harmful LDL-cholesterol and reduce blood stickiness to prevent unwanted clotting. They also have a beneficial action on bone, boosting formation of new bone and reducing absorption of old bone.

HOW MUCH YOU NEED 2.25mg to 50mg isoflavones daily. 60 grams of soy protein provides 45mg isoflavones.

RESEARCH A study involving over a hundred post-menopausal women showed that isoflavones significantly reduced the number of hot flushes experienced per day. By the 12th week of treatment, women taking soy had a 45% reduction in hot flushes versus only 30% with placebo.

Based on evidence from over 50 independent studies, the US Food and Drug Administration (FDA) have authorised health claims on food labels that "A diet low in saturated fat and cholesterol, and which includes 25g soya protein per day, can significantly reduce the risk of coronary heart disease".

A daily intake of 2.25mg isoflavones has been shown to significantly increase bone mineral content and density in the lumber spine and to protect against spinal bone loss and osteoporosis.

Isoflavones may also play an important role in protecting against breast and prostate cancers.

SIDE EFFECTS/SAFETY Isoflavones are a beneficial dietary component, and high intakes among men, women and children appear to have no obvious adverse effects.

WHAT TO LOOK FOR WHEN SELECTING A SUPPLEMENT Select a product that provides a guaranteed amount of isoflavones (eg 20mg genistein, 15mg daidzin, 4mg glycitin per 40mg isoflavones).

May be combined with Black Cohosh for additional benefit.

5HTP

WHAT IT IS 5-HTP stands for 5-hydroxy-tryptophan. It is derived from an amino acid, tryptophan, and commercial products are obtained from the seed pods of a West African plant, Griffonia simplicifolia.

WHAT IT DOES 5-HTP is converted into a brain communication chemical, serotonin, (5-hydroxy-triptamine or 5HT) which helps to lift mood and also helps to reduce food cravings in people who are depressed. Serotonin also helps to produce feelings of calm and contentment and may influence the body's biorhythms to help normalise the sleep/wake cycle.

5HTP is used to treat depression, anxiety, panic attacks, insomnia, obesity and poor concentration. It may also help people with migraine, fibromyalgia or eating disorders.

FOOD SOURCES Tryptophan, the amino acid from which 5-HTP is made in the body, is found in:

- chicken, meat and dairy products.

HOW MUCH YOU NEED Controversial. Some researchers claim 5-HTP can only be safely used as a nutritional supplement at up to 100 milligrams (mg) per day. Others suggest higher intakes of 150mg to 300mg daily (divided into three doses) for up to three months. Best taken on an empty stomach.

DEFICIENCY Uncertain, but lack of serotonin has been linked with depression, anxiety, over eating and bulimia, obsessive-compulsive behaviour, phobias, premenstrual syndrome, migraines

RESEARCH Several small studies have found 5-HTP is as effective as antidepressant drugs in reducing low mood, anxiety and insomnia.

One study suggests 5-HTP may help people with fibromyalgia. When 50 people with the condition took either 100mg 5-HTP or a placebo 3 times daily for a month, those taking active treatment had significant improvements in pain, stiffness, anxiety, sleep and fatigue.

Studies have suggested that taking 5-HTP supplements helps overweight people feel fuller, eat less calories and lose more weight than those taking an inactive placebo, as they felt less hungry and were less interested in food.

SIDE EFFECTS/SAFETY Side effects are uncommon but can include headache, nasal congestion, nausea, daytime sleepiness, nightmares and constipation.

May cause drowsiness, so should not be used if driving or operating heavy machinery.

Should only be used under medical supervision if you have a long-term health problem requiring medical treatment. Some experts have suggested it is contra-indicated or should only be used with caution in many common conditions including cardiovascular problems, autoimmune diseases, lung problems, cancer and anorexia.

5-HTP should not be used if you are taking anti-depressants, weight loss drugs, anti-Parkinson drugs, hypnotics (sleepigng tablets), antibiotics, cancer treatments, antihistamines and cold medications, alcohol - allow at least six hours between drinking alcohol and 5-HTP.

Do not take during pregnancy or breastfeeding as its effects have not been studied.

WHAT TO LOOK FOR WHEN SELECTING A SUPPLEMENT Researchers have found impurities in some 5-HTP supplements, and you may want to select a supplement that has been verified as "Peak X free".

Index

The Essential Guide to Vitamins, Minerals and Supplements

Dr Sarah Brewer

Section One: Essential Nutritional Information 7-22

Section Two: The most important Vitamins 25-41

Section Three: The most important Minerals 43-56

Section Four:
The most important Oils 59-60

What you need to know about

Section Five:
The most important Herbal supplements 63-72

What you need to know about

Section Six:
The other important food supplements 75-84

What you need to know about

NOTES

NOTES